Christians and Bioethics

Christians and Bioethics

Edited by

FRASER WATTS

To the people of the church of
St Edward King and Martyr
Cambridge

Published in Great Britain in 2000 by
Society for Promoting Christian Knowledge
Holy Trinity Church
Marylebone Road
London NW1 4DU

Bible quotations are from the *Revised Standard Version of the Bible* © 1971 and 1952,
and the *New International Version* © 1973, 1978, 1984 (by the International Bible
Society, published by Hodder & Stoughton).

British Library Cataloguing-in-Publication Data
A catalogue record for this book is available from the British Library

ISBN 0–281–05194–1

Typeset by Wilmaset Ltd, Birkenhead, Wirral
Printed in Great Britain by The Cromwell Press, Trowbridge, Wiltshire

Contents

Preface

Biotechnology is advancing at a bewildering rate. Almost every week, new possibilities seem to open up. On the day that I am writing this Preface, the newspaper has a story about a group of American scientists who are now ready to create a simple new organism from artificial DNA. Unusually, they have also announced that they will not go ahead with this for the time being, to allow opportunity for discussion of the ethical issues raised.

We urgently need good public discussion of the possibilities afforded by biotechnology. Christians have an important contribution to make to that discussion because the Christian faith provides a clear set of values from which to approach the difficult questions raised. However, before Christians can make their contribution, they themselves need to grapple with these complex issues. This book is intended to help them to do that. I hope it offers a clear and readable guide to some of the most urgent current issues in bioethics, from a distinctively Christian vantage point.

The book began as a series of lectures given at in the church of St Edward King and Martyr, in the centre of Cambridge, where I am Vicar-Chaplain. As I listened to those excellent lectures, I realized that they deserved to be made available to a much wider audience, and I am pleased that this book does so. I am grateful to my Cambridge friends and colleagues who took the trouble, first to give their lectures at St Edward's, and then to prepare them for publication. I am also grateful for the challenge and opportunity of my ministry at St Edward's, which led me to bring these important issues forward for wider discussion and debate. This book is dedicated, in gratitude, to the people of St Edward's, Cambridge.

Fraser Watts

Queens' College Cambridge   *St Paul's Day, 1999*

About the Contributors

The Reverend Dr Tim Appleton is an independent Fertility Counsellor.

Professor Derek Burke, CBE, was formerly Vice-Chancellor of the University of East Anglia, and Chairman of the Advisory Committee on Novel Foods and Processes from 1989 to 1997.

The Reverend Professor Michael Langford was formerly Professor of Philosophy and Professor of Medical Ethics at the Memorial University of Newfoundland.

The Reverend Dr John Polkinghorne, KBE, FRS, was formerly Professor of Mathematical Physics in the University of Cambridge, and President of Queens' College, Cambridge.

Dr Michael Rees is an Assistant Professor in the Department of Urology at the Medical College of Ohio, currently on sabbatical as a Fellow in Transplantation at the Department of Surgery in the University of Cambridge.

The Reverend Dr Fraser Watts is Starbridge Lecturer in Theology and Natural Science in the University of Cambridge, Fellow of Queens' College, and Vicar-Chaplain of St Edward King and Martyr, Cambridge.

CHAPTER ONE

Approaches to Bioethics

Fraser Watts

We live in a world in which biotechnology is developing at a bewildering rate. The possibilities are increasing faster than most of us can assimilate. This book considers some of them, such as the rapid development of genetically engineering food, the cloning of the first animals and the related possibilities of using 'engineered' animals to grow organs for transplant surgery, and the many ways in which medicine is now able to assist human reproduction.

Not everything that is possible is also right. The ethical challenge at the present time is to see which of the possible (and soon to be possible) applications of biotechnology should actually be used. Because the issues are so new, and progress is so rapid, we are not ready to answer these questions. There simply has not yet been enough informed, ethically sensitive discussion among society at large for a consensus to emerge about what is and is not right. Making ethical judgements is a social business. It depends on the collective judgement of an ethical community, and with biotechnology we do not yet have the kind of collective ethical judgements we need.

That makes things very difficult for everyone involved, especially for the scientists who are developing new possibilities. Scientists are as concerned about ethical proprieties as much as anyone else, indeed more than most. However, it is difficult for them to decide what research and practical developments are appropriate if society has not given them a way of telling where the ethical dividing line comes. How can politicians regulate the use of biotechnology on behalf of society if society has no implicit ethical consensus?

Developing such a consensus is made difficult by the rapid

development of biotechnology, but it is also made difficult by the fact that we do not quite know 'where we are coming from' in making ethical judgements. We live in a pluralistic society, in which there are all sorts of approaches to ethical questions. Up to a point that is helpful, because it safeguards against the totalitarian approach to ethical issues that can arise in a society in which one particular ideology, religious or otherwise, reigns supreme and unchallenged. However, pluralism also has its dangers. When pluralism has reached the point at which ethical discussion has become completely fragmented and incoherent, it may be difficult for society to develop any kind of ethical response to urgent questions such as those posed by biotechnology.

It is in this context that Christians find themselves. Religious traditions, including Christianity, provide one of the fundamental frameworks in which ethical discussion can take place. They provide the concepts and principles out of which bioethics can be developed. In this sense, society badly needs the coherent and principled approach to bioethics that Christianity is capable of offering. This is widely recognized in the way in which religious representatives are appointed to ethical committees.

However, Christians, like everyone else, are struggling with the rapid pace of biotechnology. It takes time and care to reflect in a Christian way on the new possibilities now before us. We cannot just read up the answers in the Bible, or turn to what past authorities had to say. All the same, that does not mean that Christianity has nothing to offer. It means that we must go back to the fundamental principles of the Christian tradition and use them to think out what is a right response to the new issues raised by biotechnology.

Ethics

Ethics is in part a matter of making judgements about the practical consequences of particular courses of action. However, that is never quite enough. In ethics, you also need the fundamental values from which possible consequences can be seen to be right or wrong. Very few of the outcomes made possible by the new biotechnology are unequivocally good or unequivocally bad. If they were, bioethics would be a much easier business than it is. Generally, there are pros and cons to be weighed up, and this is where an ethical framework, such as the Christian one, is especially important.

However, having an ethical framework does not mean that discussion of consequences is redundant. Sometimes people imagine that religious traditions such as Christianity can simply tell them what is right or wrong, without having to get involved in any detailed consideration of the likely consequences of particular actions. I do not believe that is so. Christian ethics arises out of the dialogue between basic principles and a rational examination of likely consequences. Both are indispensable to the ethical task.

Philosophers have often discussed these matters in terms of the relationship between what 'is' the case, and what 'ought' to be the case. There is a clear distinction to be made between 'is' and 'ought', but I suggest that ethics needs both. It needs the best factual judgements we are able to make about what is the case, and especially about what would happen if we take certain lines of action. However, those factual judgements need to be considered in the light of the basic values that guide our judgements about what ought to happen. Ethics requires both 'is' and 'ought'. The two can be distinguished, but both are required, and they need to become intertwined in our judgements about what is right.

In considering issues in bioethics, there is an important distinction to be made between positive and negative objectives of new developments in biotechnology. There is, for example, a very important difference between the positive aim of seeking to improve the human race and the negative one of seeking to eliminate particular diseases or defects. Many people feel that negative objectives raise fewer ethical problems than positive ones, and that we should confine ourselves to objectives such as treating disease, and not go beyond that and try to make things better and better.

One reason why this distinction is important is that value judgements are much more difficult to make when it comes to improving the human race than when we are simply remedying defects. There are many illnesses and other related health problems about which there is no disagreement. Cancer, for example, is a great scourge and a source of incredible suffering and distress. Medicine has always sought to eliminate such obvious maladies as far as it is able, and I see no problem with that. It is certainly a central part of the tradition that Christians have inherited from Jesus to seek to heal the sick. There seems just no doubt that this is desirable.

However, the distinction between positive and negative aims is not always as clear as might be supposed. For example, there is a fine line between seeking to raise the general intellectual stock of the human race and trying to eliminate mental handicap. Also, as Tim Appleton indicates in his chapter on reproductive medicine, it is hard to know whether enabling couples who wish to have children to do so represents a general improvement in the human race, or a remedying of the disease of infertility. The boundary between removing illness and handicap and making more general improvements can be a shifting one.

An anxiety that frequently recurs in discussion of bioethics is about the 'slippery slope'. The fear is that if we begin by making modest use of the possibilities opened up by the new biotechnology, that will inevitably lead to much wider applications later. People fear that we will end up going too far. The conclusion that is usually drawn from the 'slippery slope' argument is that it is best not even to begin, in case things get out of hand.

There is some obvious sense in this argument. It is probably correct that taking modest steps now will make it more likely that bigger steps will be taken in the future. However, it does not make it inevitable. It can equally well be argued that taking modest steps will enable us to see more clearly, and with the benefit of greater experience, just how far down a particular path of biotechnology we wish to go. It seems better to look at each development in biotechnology on its merits, rather than to refrain from taking one step that is clearly desirable for fear of where it might lead.

Nature

One of the most fundamental issues that arises in discussing these matters is what degree of respect we should have for nature, for how things are. Many people share the idea that nature is in some sense sacred, and that we should not be 'monkeying around' with it in the way that biotechnology appears to be doing.

It is hard to be quite sure where this feeling comes from that nature should not be interfered with. Partly it seems to hark back to the religious thinking of earlier ages, in which it was often assumed that God had created the world perfect. If you take that view, it follows that any kind of interference with nature is bound to make it worse. However, the imperfections of the world are very apparent, and it is difficult to sustain the idea that nature is incapable of improvement. It does not seem to have been made perfect. Christians might also note that there is little support for that idea in the teaching of Jesus.

The idea of perfection was also linked to the belief that nature had never changed. For example, it was thought that all species had existed from the outset, and that they had existed in such a perfect balance and ecology that no changes in any species, or in the relationship between them, had ever been required. But that was before Darwin. There is now almost universal acceptance of some form of the theory of evolution. We may still not understand everything about exactly how evolution has occurred, but the grounds for accepting some form of evolution are utterly compelling. The world *has* changed. Its present state cannot be equated either with an original state, or with a perfect one.

The idea that nature should not be interfered with also sometimes seems to have its roots in a pantheistic identification of nature with what is sacred. Rather than saying that God created nature exactly as it is, you can cut out the creation by God, and say simply that nature is in some sense divine, is actually God. That leads to the conclusion that in interfering with nature we are interfering directly with God. In many ways it has been valuable in our time to have a growing sense of the sacredness of nature. It has helped us to treat it in a more responsible way. However, this welcome spirit of reverence for nature need not be based on the extreme idea that nature is God, and it does not necessarily prohibit any attempt at the modification of nature.

Certainly, we should be alert to the possibility that in trying to improve things in some ways we will make them worse in others. Medicine has long had to grapple with that problem. There is much 'iatrogenic' disease, illness brought on by medical treatment itself. We cannot focus solely on the good we hope to do and shut our eyes to the harm we may also inadvertently do. However, there is no reason why we should be so scared of inadvertent harm that we do nothing at all. Human beings have always tried to make their world better. We have never turned our back on all possible improvements for fear of doing harm, and there is no clear reason why we should do so now.

People respond by saying that the consequences of biotechnology are too difficult to assess. It is felt that we simply cannot calculate the harm that may result, for example, from genetically engineered food. Of course, there is always an element of unpredictability about the consequences of any new innovation. Medicine has always had to cope with not really knowing the consequences of new treatments until they have been introduced. The proper response to this unpredictability, I suggest, is to gather all relevant information, make the best judgement possible about the likely consequences, and decide on that basis whether or not to proceed. I do not think it is right either blithely to disregard potential harm, or to be cowed by the problem of unpredictability into doing nothing.

Another objection to modifying nature is that in doing so we would be 'playing God' in a way that would be presumptuous and wrong. It is an objection to biotechnology advanced, for example, by Paul Ramsey, one of the most distinguished Christian thinkers of recent decades to have wrestled with issues in medical ethics. However, it is not clear that Christianity says that any attempt to modify nature is 'playing God'. That would only follow if we saw our attempted refinement of nature as equivalent to the work of God as creator. That would be a very strange thing for a Christian to think.

There is a huge difference between our creative activity and that of God. Christians have often tried to characterize the distinctive nature of God's creative work by saying that he created 'out of nothing'. We do not do that. All human creative work depends on taking what we find in the world and rearranging it. Scientists might talk, for example, about creating an artificial organism 'from scratch', but that is not at all like God creating 'out of nothing'. The key point is that God's creative work is free and wholly unconstrained.

The idea that we are perhaps playing God seems to come from thinking about God's role as creator in too anthropomorphic terms. We imagine that God is like some glorified human being, imagine that he made the world much as we might have tried to do. We then think of our attempted improvements on nature as being like the work of God, and condemn them on that basis. It is an odd line of argument that has its roots in thinking of God, in the first place, as like some kind of human being.

Persons

Though some of the issues raised by the new biotechnology are concerned with the non-human aspects of creation (and issues about genetically engineered food, discussed in Derek Burke's chapter, are perhaps the hottest topic of this kind at present), many of the new issues are concerned with human beings. There are distinctive issues here. We might feel that it was acceptable to make changes to the rest of creation, but that human beings were in some way 'off limits', and that we should not try and change ourselves.

It is always difficult to maintain a balanced view of how human beings relate to the rest of creation, and tempting either to exaggerate or to minimize the differences between ourselves and other species. Neither extreme is plausible. Clearly we have much in common with the animal world from which we have evolved, and virtually everything which seems to be 'special' about human beings has its roots in other higher primates. However, there are attributes which have developed in us to a much higher degree than in any other creatures known to us, such as our moral sense, our reflective self-consciousness, our facility with language, our capacity for relationships. Human beings really are different from other species, but the differences are often ones of degree, not absolute differences. Not that these distinctive human attributes are an unmitigated blessing; they enable us to do a great deal of good, but they also enable us to do more harm than perhaps any other species.

· One argument that is sometimes advanced against trying to modify the human race, or radically improve its lot, rests on the assumption that it is in the nature of humanity that we are (a) flawed and (b) very diverse. It is then argued that nothing should be done that in any way minimizes either our diversity or our failings as a species. I do not find that argument convincing. Perhaps a version of humanity that was no longer imperfect would not be the humanity we know. However, the question which is being posed here is completely hypothetical. We simply do not have the choice between making ourselves a perfect species or leaving ourselves imperfect. The ways in which we can improve our lot are becoming increasingly significant, but no good comes from exaggerating them. Neither should we confuse what we may actually be able to do in the foreseeable future with what there is no prospect of our ever being able to do. Bioethics is in no position to make us perfect.

It is also true that there is great variety in the human race, and that if we were able to eliminate our faults, then humanity would be less diverse. The resulting species might be in some sense less interesting than we are now. However, it is again important not to exaggerate what we can do, or are likely to be able to do. Bioethics does not seem to hold out the potential of making all human beings near-identical.

A more significant concern, in my view, is how human bio-technology might affect our attitudes to people who have particular characteristics. This arises most clearly with genetic engineering. For example, a programme of genetic engineering that aimed to eliminate a particular characteristic from the human race would almost inevitably affect attitudes to people with that characteristic. People with mental handicaps are an interesting example. Many parents of people with mental handicaps find it particularly rewarding to be the parents of such people. They might even feel that life was impoverished if they did not have that opportunity. Similarly, innovations in reproductive medicine may result in society taking a negative view of those who remained infertile, and so on.

There probably really is a link between respect for people who possess certain attributes, and refraining from attempting to modify those attributes. Programmes of modifications could easily increase stigmatization. There are perhaps particular reasons why Christians should be concerned about this. The Christian tradition can be very helpful in enabling people to see how good can come out of suffering and imperfection, and this is rooted in the redemption that came out of Christ's suffering on the cross. This can lead, in turn, to our treating people with handicaps with greater respect than might otherwise be the case. At very least, these are matters that need to be considered when any particular applications of biotechnology arise.

There are also particular issues about attitudes to babies raised by the advances in reproductive medicine discussed in Tim Appleton's chapter. Babies who are conceived in highly artificial ways might be regarded differently from those conceived more naturally. In the most extreme case, this would be true of human clones, as John Polkinghorne indicates. None of us would want to think we had been born just to be a clone of someone else. It is worth noting here that God has apparently refrained from making us embodiments of his perfection, but has given us the freedom to depart from that. We are not clones of God, and neither would we wish to be clones of another human being.

In all discussions about human bioethics, it is important to hold on to the principle we are 'persons'. All decisions about what is appropriate in human biotechnology need to be based on an adequate understanding of what it is to be a person, and what is appropriate for persons. This leads back to the distinctive attributes of human beings to which I have already referred. We are, in large measure, conscious, responsible, relational creatures, and it is a fundamental ethical principle that we should try to behave as such ourselves, and treat each other similarly. In making ethical judgements, in reproductive medicine for example, we need to remember that we are talking about the reproduction of persons. Decisions about the appropriateness of euthanasia or assisted suicide also need to be based on a clear judgement about how far someone is still a person.

We tend to think of persons as having 'rights' in some special sense. (I will not enter here into the question of whether animals should also be regarded as having rights.) People are coming to have an increasingly strong sense of their rights, their right to have children, their right to an organ for transplantation, their right to die, and so on. Interestingly, the use of the language of rights is not confined to liberal perspectives. Conservative, anti-abortion views are sometimes also presented in terms of the right of a foetus to life.

Though rights are an important aspect of persons and our dealings with one another, I do not believe that it is appropriate to reduce human ethics entirely to a matter of rights. Rights need to be considered in relation to responsibilities and more general considerations about what is appropriate to persons. The distinctive issues about bioethics that arise with human beings should not be narrowed to just a matter of rights.

The Christian Approach

So far, I have looked at approaches to bioethics that, for the most part, would make as much sense to non-Christians as to Christians. I believe there is much to be said for Christians approaching things in that spirit, as Michael Langford explains in his chapter. However, I have also said the bioethics debate needs the coherent, principled approach that the Christian tradition can offer. So what is the particular Christian contribution?

One key Christian idea is that we have been given stewardship of creation. It is consistent with the many stories of Jesus about a master going away and leaving his property in the hands of stewards. The question to which this leads is what kind of stewardship has been exercised. Leaving everything as it is, and putting nature in mothballs, is not necessarily the best approach. The steward who hid the talents his master had left him, rather than risking investing them, was chastised for his lack of courage, rather than commended for his overriding wish to preserve what he had been entrusted with (see Matthew 25.14–30).

This concept of stewardship leads on to the further idea that we have come to share in God's work of creation. The degree of influence over the natural world that we now possess means that we can see ourselves as 'co-creators' with God, even though, as I have already emphasized, we cannot presume to be the kind of ultimate source of creation that Christians believe God to be. God's creative work is a continuing one, not a single 'once for all' action, and we have the opportunity to share in God's continuing creation. The interesting paradox is that we are both part of creation, but also now in some sense co-creators with God. We are thus, in Philip Hefner's helpful phrase, 'created co-creators'. That implies that we should approach our stewardship of creation responsibly, trying to discern where we are acting in accordance with God's creative purposes.

Of course, alongside the idea of stewardship there is, within the Judeo-Christian tradition, a stronger version of the role of humanity in relation to nature, that we have been given 'dominion' over it. This idea comes from the verse in Genesis that says, 'Let us make man in our image, after our likeness; and let them have dominion over the fish of the sea...' (1.26 RSV). This notion of dominion gives even less support for the idea that nature should not be interfered with. However, many have pointed out the abuses to which too strong a notion of dominion has led. I would prefer to see our relationship to nature in terms of stewardship rather than dominion, but even the 'softer' notion of stewardship gives no support to the idea that nature should be left absolutely alone.

Seeing ourselves as created co-creators provides a helpful framework within which to approach issues in bioethics in a specifically Christian way. It does not prevent us from doing anything at all to modify nature, but neither does it imply that we can do anything we like. It implies that any modifications of nature that we undertake should be ones that are consistent with what we discern to be the creative purposes of God. Of course, that is not a straightforward criterion to apply in practice, but it leads us to ask the right kind of questions.

It is a way of approaching things that stands in sharp contrast to all attempts to narrow the framework within which bioethics is approached. There are currently various attempts to adopt a narrow approach. One is in terms of consequences. If bioethics is approached in a purely practical spirit, and we only ask whether a particular development will do more good or harm, questions become much easier to answer. An approach exclusively in terms of rights is another superficially attractive but narrow framework.

The appeal of narrow frameworks for approaching ethical questions is obvious. It makes them much easier to resolve. The Christian approach, as I have suggested, is based on the question of whether our proposed actions are consistent with God's creative purposes. That is a very broad framework to adopt. Indeed, because there is no larger reality than God, there is perhaps no broader perspective from which to look at things than that of God's purposes. Perhaps one of the key contributions Christians will want to make to the current debates in bioethics is to keep a broad and open perspective on the magnitude of the issues involved, but to do that without excessive timidity. I hope this book will help people to look at some of the pressing current issues in bioethics in that spirit.

Suggested Reading

An influential early book that set out a conservative position was:

P. Ramsey, *Fabricated Man: The Ethics of Genetic Control*. New Haven, Yale University Press, 1970.

There is a useful discussion of Ramsey's position, and the more pragmatic position of Joseph Fletcher to which it was a response, in Dyson's chapter in

A.E. Dyson and J. Harris (eds), *Ethics and Biotechnology*. London, Routledge, 1994.

A very accessible introduction to bioethics for Christians is:

G. Meilaender, *Bioethics: A Primer for Christians*. Carlisle, Paternoster Press, 1996.

Other more penetrating books on Christian bioethics are:

C. Deane-Drummond, *Theology and Biotechnology: Implications for a New Science*. London, Geoffrey Chapman, 1997.

J. Harris, *Wonderwoman and Superman: The Ethics of Biotechnology*. Oxford, Oxford University Press. 1994.

J. Mahoney, *Bioethics and Belief*. London, Sheed & Ward, 1984.

The following are useful edited collections:

J.F. Kilner, N.M. de S. Cameron and D.L. Schiedermayer (eds), *Bioethics and the Future of Medicine: A Christian Appraisal*. Grand Rapids, Eerdmans, 1995.

A.L. Verhey and S.E. Lammers, *Theological Voices in Medical Ethics*. Grand Rapids, Eerdmans, 1993.

On particular issues about human persons, see:

J. Habgood, *Being a Person: Where Science and Faith Meet*. London, Hodder & Stoughton, 1998.

For the concept of created co-creators, see:

P. Hefner, *The Human Factor: Evolution, Culture and Religion*. Minneapolis, Fortress Press, 1993.

A broad range of issues in medical ethics has been considered in the *Journal of Medical Ethics*, London, Society of Medical Ethics, 1975–.

CHAPTER TWO

Cloning: After Dolly

John Polkinghorne

D olly must be the most famous sheep in the world. We have all seen her photograph. I am told that she appears to enjoy her fame, coming forward to greet visitors when they arrive to see her.

Two things make Dolly famous. One is that she is an artificially induced clone, genetically identical to a previously existing sheep and made so by the skilful operations of the scientists at the Roslin Institute, who manipulated and implanted the embryo that gave rise to her birth. The other thing that makes Dolly famous is the way in which this was done. Almost all the genetic material in a cell (the DNA) is contained in the cell's nucleus. The Roslin scientists took the nucleus from a cell obtained from the udder of an adult sheep and implanted it in an egg cell whose original nucleus had been removed. Such acts of nuclear transplantation had been performed successfully before, but only using nuclei from embryonic cells. At such an early stage of development the DNA is still omnicompetent, capable of generating the growth of a whole animal. Later in development, specialization sets in. Cells become differentiated into heart cells, liver cells, etc. The whole of the genetic material is still there, but most of it is switched off and only the genes relative to that particular type of cell are active. It had been thought that this differentiation was irreversible, so that an udder cell could only give rise to more udder cells. The scientists at Roslin discovered how to reverse this. As Dolly showed, it became possible to produce a clone of a mature adult. It was this fact that gave rise to so much scientific surprise and public interest.

Nuclear transplantation is not the only way of producing a clone. An alternative procedure is embryo-splitting, the division of an early embryo, at a stage where it has comparatively few cells, into two separate clusters. This is a process that sometimes occurs naturally, resulting in identical twins. Because there is a small amount of genetic material (called mitochondrial DNA) that is present in a cell outside the nucleus, embryo-splitting produces a truly perfect clone, while clones made by nuclear transfer will have different mitochondrial DNA and so have some small genetic differences from each other. However, embryo splitting cannot be used to produce the clone of an adult. It is a procedure that could only generate very few copies, while nuclear transplantation could, in principle, generate as many copies as were desired.

The work at Roslin was undertaken for serious and responsible purposes. It is possible to modify animals genetically in a small and specific way with the result that, for example, their milk then contains a protein (such as a clotting factor for human blood needed by haemophiliacs) which is of therapeutic value to human beings. Such procedures are difficult and only occasionally successful. The resulting animals are of very considerable value, both financially and medically. If it were possible to multiply them by cloning, that would be a procedure of considerable significance. Of course, it would also be possible in the same way to multiply naturally occurring individual animals that had highly desirable characteristics – Derby winners, for instance.

In the popular mind and media, the furore about Dolly was not generated by thoughts about animal cloning. It was the possible use of the same technique to make human clones that caught the lurid imaginations of many commentators. A great deal of the discussion was apocalyptic and fantastic. The ugly spectre of eugenics was raised, with scenarios such as the State production of 'standard issue' worker clones like the proles of Aldous Huxley's chilling novel, *Brave New World*. The notion was discussed of powerful dictators, or the immensely rich, clutching at some kind of self-propagation through having clones made of themselves, like Adolf Hitler in the film, *The Boys from Brazil*. More touchingly, but quite fallaciously, it was suggested that the bereaved might find a 'replacement' of a lost parent, or lost child, by the birth of a clone, as if a strict genetic determinism reigns and persons were no more than their genes. In fact, of course, such clones would be new people. A clone of Hitler might have grown up to be an insigificant Austrian house-painter.

Despite the fantastic character of much of the initial hype following the birth of Dolly, there are serious ethical issues to consider relating to cloning. All scientific discoveries bring in their train a number of technological possibilities for their exploitation and use. Some of these applications will be valuable; some will be harmful. Society needs to be able, as far as it possibly can, to choose the good and refuse the bad. The process of discrimination will be likely to be conducted better if much of the thinking is undertaken before there is the pressure exerted for hasty decision by the existence of the technology already 'on the shelf'. In making decisions of this kind, scientific knowledge has to have wisdom added to it. The scientists, as scientists, have no monopoly in access to ethical insight. Society at large has an indispensable role to play and the great religious traditions are reservoirs of wisdom in moral matters.

Reproductive and Therapeutic Cloning

In thinking about the use of the nuclear transplantation technique, it is important to recognize that there are two quite distinct possible fields of application, reproductive cloning and therapeutic cloning.

Reproductive cloning would be the exact analogue of Dolly, involving the creation of a cloned embryo which was then implanted in a woman's womb to develop to term and the birth of a human clone. This procedure was what the initial fantastic speculations were concerned with and its possibility has rightly resulted in a great deal of unease among responsible commentators. The House of Commons Select Committee dealing with scientific and medical matters issued a report very soon after the news of Dolly had become public, stating that there should be no creation of 'experimental human beings'. Reproductive human cloning would, in fact, be illegal in Britain under the provisions of the Human Fertilisation and Embryology Act.

Therapeutic cloning would not result in the implantation or birth of a human clone but it would involve the growing of cellular human tissue of specific kinds. Two broad purposes could be fulfilled by such a procedure. One would be as an important tool for the scientific study of medically significant cellular processes, such as ageing or malignancy. The other would be to generate genetically compatible tissue (not at risk of immunological rejection in the patient) for the treatment of certain conditions, such as in Parkinsonism or for the repair of damaged heart muscle. The ethical issues here should be recognized as being different from those stemming from the possibility of cloning of human individuals. In Britain, such procedures would be legal under licence from the Human Fertility and Embryology Authority, during the fourteen-day period of embryonic age during which research is permitted, if the Secretary of State were to make an appropriate order to this effect.

Theological and Ethical Issues

Clear thinking and informed debate are necessary if we are to make good decisions about the possibilities that rapidly developing genetic science sets before us. Among the theological and ethical issues to be considered are, first, people's concern that we may be '*playing God*'. Many feel unease about current developments because they fear that certain natural barriers are being crossed that it is dangerous or impious for humanity to transgress. Genetics is concerned with 'the stuff of life', and should we not hold back from interference with it? Religious people may want to express this reserve by questioning whether it is not the case that creatures are in danger of attempting to usurp the prerogatives of the Creator.

On the other hand, human beings have long been intervening in nature to change the character of purely natural process. Medicine and surgery are obvious examples of such interventions. A religious person can see this activity, when it is devoted to serious and beneficial ends, as an appropriate use of God-given human capacities, rather than an inappropriate attempt to rival the Creator. Nevertheless, not everything that can be done, should be done. There is the possibility of the misuse of human powers. In the treatment of human disease, there is currently an agreement that it is ethically permissible to use somatic gene therapy (that is, changing the genetic character of some cells in the body in a way that carries no consequences beyond the person so treated, and in order to remedy a genetic defect), but there is a moratorium on germ-line gene therapy (that is to say, interventions that would propagate to future generations). In part, this distinction arises

16

because of a great uncertainty about the safety of the long-term consequences of germ-line changes. However, there are some who would oppose germ-line intervention for fundamental ethical reasons based on the moral unacceptablity of changing human nature in this way, with all its potentiality for eugenic manipulation.

Those who use the discourse of *animal* rights (as opposed to a human duty of respect to other forms of life), will see a high degree of moral equivalence between animals and human beings, claiming that nothing should be done to animals that is not for their individual good. They will oppose *animal cloning*, regarding the sort of experiments that led to Dolly as being unacceptable. Those who believe that there is an ethically justifiable degree of instrumental use of animals (illustrated, for example, by the eating of meat) will not take so absolute a view. They will, of course, wish such activity to be controlled by safeguards relating to animal welfare, minimization of suffering (which should bear a propor-tionate relationship to potential human benefit), and seriousness of the purpose for which the activities are undertaken. The Roslin experiments can certainly be held to fulfil these criteria. In fact, cloned animals like Dolly are of such value and significance that they can be expected to be accorded the highest standards of care in their subsequent lives.

The European Bioethics Commission called for the banning of reproductive human cloning, asserting as an argument that *every human being is entitled to their own individual and unique genetic identity*. While the conclusion may be valid, the character of the reasoning offered in its support is highly questionable. What about identical twins? They are genetically indistinguishable, but no one doubts that they are two distinct and unique persons. The rights of one are not threatened by the existence of the other. Once again, one must protest that, though we are constrained by our genetic inheritance, we are not determined by it.

Another concern is *safety*. In the experiments that led to Dolly, 277 attempts at nuclear transplantation were made, resulting in only 29 implantable embryos and leading to only one completed pregnancy and birth – Dolly. Some other forms of embryonic manipulations are known to lead to enhanced rates of defective pregnancy and malformed births. There is some uncertainty about what 'age' Dolly will prove to be, her birth age or the age of the ewe that provided the nucleus. Will cloned animals show enhanced susceptibilities to cancer and other diseases because their genes are already 'aged'?

Even if human reproductive cloning were considered ethically acceptable on other grounds, there would still be very severe questions about the safety of the procedure and the degree of wastage that could occur as part of it. These questions could only be settled, first by extensive animal investigations and then experiments with human subjects. The ethical unacceptability of such experiments is what the Select Committee asserted in its report, a conclusion accepted by the Health Minister, Tessa Jowell.

Many of the reasons hypothetically advanced for human reproductive cloning, such as replacement of lost kin and the perpetuation of particular individuals, are not only fallacious because they fail to acknowledge the uniqueness of every human person, in whatever way their genetic endowment might relate to that of another, but they are also totally ethically unacceptable because of their *instrumental treatment of the new human being* thus brought into existence. Every child that is born is to be valued for his or her own sake and not as the replacement or perpetuation of another. As Kant and many other ethical writers have emphasized, human beings are always ends and never means to some other end. It would be a crippling psychological burden for a child to learn that they were brought into the world to be the substitute for someone else.

A similar morally repugnant instrumentality lies behind eugenic proposals for the bringing about of persons whose genetic make-up has been carefully crafted to the specifications of someone else. Such 'designer babies' would represent the ethically unacceptable commodification of children.

Nuclear transplantation could be used to bring about genetically related children in circumstances where neither natural conception nor normal IVF treatment were possible. As an extreme example, a lesbian couple could generate a child from the ennucleated egg of one of the women and the nucleus from a cell of the other. One must ask the ethical question whether there are not limits that need to be set to fulfilling a couple's desire for genetically related children. IVF treatment involves enabling a natural process, which would normally take place within the body, to take place outside the body because the normal course of nature is impeded for some reason. Nuclear transplantation is a radically unnatural process. It could never take place without direct scientific intervention. There is much ethical debate about what is the *relationship of the moral to the natural*, but there will certainly be those who would wish to draw this distinction between enabling the natural and facilitating the unnatural, at least in relation to human fertility.

There are a number of possible ways in which the nuclear transplantation technique might find application in the *treatment of human disease*. Some of these have already been outlined in the definition of therapeutic cloning. The degree of moral difficulty felt in assessing the ethical character of the options thus presented will depend upon an assessment of the moral status that the human embryo possesses from fertilization onwards. Some Christian opinion, including the official position of the Roman Catholic Church, affords to the embryo the full moral status of a human person. In that case, any genetic manipulation of the embryo will be considered unacceptable.

The Warnock Committee, whose Report led eventually to the setting up of the Human Fertilisation and Embryology Authority with power to license certain embryo procedures during the first fourteen days (a period linked to the onset of differentiation and the appearance of 'the primitive streak'), did not take so stringent a view. It accorded a deep ethical respect to the human embryo, on the basis of its potential to develop into a human being, but it did not equate it to a person. This is the ethical basis on which the HFEA was given the power that would enable it to license therapeutic cloning within the fourteen-day limit.

There are some who take a position intermediate between these two extremities. They are happy about embryo work in the fourteen-day period that is conducted with the primary intent of assisting procreation, and even for 'spare' embryos, not needed for implantation, to be made available for research. However, they are not happy with the idea of creating human embryos with the primary intent of their being used for research purposes. They feel this is an undesirable degree of instrumental use. Presumably they may feel similar reservations about such work done with therapeutic intentions. Certainly, any such proposal will have to make clear what is the source of the eggs which are to be ennucleated. After all, human eggs are in short supply for fertility purposes. However, once a therapeutically valuable cell line was established, its multiplication could then continue without the need to use further eggs.

A second possible application of the nuclear transplantation technique arises in the case of certain rare but severe diseases that originate from defects in the mitochondrial DNA, present in the cell material outside the nucleus. Nuclear transplantation could, in principle, offer a way of combating these diseases. The nucleus of a fertilized egg would be removed from the presence of the defective mitochondrial DNA and implanted in an enunciated cell with healthy mitochondrial DNA. The resulting embryo would then be implanted in the womb for normal gestation. The procedure would not be legal in Britain under present law, because of the ban on implanting manipulated embryos. It would, however, offer what is perhaps the only conceivable way of treating these serious conditions. The result would not strictly speaking be a clone, for the nuclear genetic endowment of the resulting child would be that of the original embryo and it would not be the same as that of any other existing human being.

Applied genetics is a rapidly developing field. It is important that the ethical character of the new technology should, as far as possible, be considered at the stage where options are still glints in the eyes of experimenters and not already practical possibilities on the shelf, pressing to be used. Many beneficial discoveries will be made but there will also be opportunities for harmful misuse. Not everything that can be done, should be done. We need a sustained dialogue between the experts (who alone can evaluate possibilities and their consequences) and the general public (who have a legitimate concern about what is being done). Christians should play their full part in helping society to make the right choices, both in the light of scientific knowledge well understood and also in the light of ethical insights carefully evaluated.

Suggested Reading

T. Peters, *Playing God?* London, Routledge, 1997.

R. Cole-Turner, *Human Cloning: Religious Perspectives.* Louisville, KY, Westminster John Knox, 1997.

CHAPTER THREE

Genetic Engineering of Food

Derek Burke

Consumers have enjoyed, over the last 20 years, a huge increase in the range and quality of the food available to them, with real decreases in food prices. The variety, the freshness and the choice available in every supermarket is now taken for granted, while the technological revolution in delivery, in stock control and in marketing is very impressive. Britain has an advanced system for food retailing, and it is the retailers that control the food chain, both backwards to the producer and forwards to the consumer. The retailers have formidable buying power and will specify precisely how a crop is to be sown, watered and harvested, what pesticides are to be used and when, and if the price is not right then they will go elsewhere! They know a lot about you and me too, for every time we shop with our customer loyalty card we are telling them what we have bought, and when, and since they know where we live and our post code is correlatable with our buying power and preferences, they know, for example, for any day, or hour, how many middle-class customers are buying that new brand of yoghurt.

So, new products are being introduced all the time, evaluated and, if not successful, discontinued. We take for granted a continuous stream of new products, and always at a very competitive price; for the fierce competition between the chains sees to that. And behind those new products lie many new processes. My point is that we now accept, and indeed expect, a very wide choice of foods at ever decreasing prices. And how does biotechnology fit into that? Well, it is one of the engines of change to provide products which are cheaper, healthier or last longer. But first a word about what biotechnology is.

Biotechnology

Biotechnology derives from three techniques discovered only in the last 20 years:

- The ability to cut and stitch DNA. Specific enzymes can be used to cut DNA into gene-sized pieces which are then inserted into bacteria. These transformed bacteria are used to amplify and separate the many different DNA pieces, which are then sequenced by a mixture of chemical and biochemical techniques. Any of these pieces can be inserted into another DNA genome.

- The ability to move DNA and genes from one organism to another and, moreover, the ability to persuade new genes to work in the new organisms. This is possible because, rather broadly, the way genes work is universal, from bacteria to human beings. These two techniques are what is called 'genetic modification'.

- The ability to modify proteins by a process termed 'protein engineering'. This involves systematic alteration of the DNA sequence which will, in turn, alter the aminoacid sequence of a protein, thus altering its properties.

Some of the applications of this new technology are obvious; growth hormone can now be made in bacteria rather than extracted from cadavers, so providing a source that is free of contamination with the agent for the Creutzfeldt-Jakob Disease, and the supply of insulin for diabetics or of interferon for patients with Hepatitis B is no longer limited. We also need to grow more food, and soon farmers will be able to use less herbicide, and lose less of their corn crop to insects, because they will be growing plants resistant to the herbicides and pests. The world's population is increasing at about 1.5 per cent per year (about 87 million per year), and is estimated to grow from its present 5.9 billion to 8 billion by 2020. In addition, loss of land to urbanization means that the amount of cultivated land supporting food production has fallen from 0.44 ha per person in 1961 to 0.26 now, and is projected to fall to 0.15 ha per person by 2050. The need for irrigation is increasing, climate is changing and as people become more prosperous, they replace plant foods with animal foods – which are less efficient in trapping solar energy.

About one half of the grain produced in Europe, North America and Russia is already used as animal feed. Critics argue that the planet's food problems are due to economic and political problems, not because we cannot grow enough. There is truth in that, and we need to do better, but I very much doubt if we shall solve all our problems that way, and it seems perverse to me to walk away from a potential substantial increase in the world's food supply.

Most of the genes that I have described so far have been what are called structural genes; genes that determine the structure of a particular protein. But recently other genes, genes that control development, have been isolated. For example, the genes that control flower shape and colour in the snapdragon. This means that we can start to alter flower shape and colour for the horticultural industry. More importantly, the genes that control the plant's response to day length have been isolated. This means that it may be possible, by modifying these genes, to produce plants that come to maturity more quickly, with a huge economic impact.

So what is biotechnology likely to do for food and crops? The most straightforward developments will be a whole series of new and improved enzymes for food processing and for the modification of existing foods, for example modification of fats by a process known as interesterification with the introduction of unsaturated fatty acids or fatty acids yielding fewer calories. A Mars bar which claims to yield fewer calories is already on sale in the US. The science is straightforward, and there seems to be little consumer concern.

There will also be many new crop products; of three general types:

- modifications of the genetic material of plants to extend their shelf life by slowing down the enzyme responsible for the breakdown of the plant cell walls, for example the new tomato, and a melon to come;

- modification of the genetic material of plants to produce novel parental lines for the production of new F1 hybrids, for example rape;

- modification of the genetic material of plants to introduce resistance to herbicides or pests, for example, soya, potatoes, cotton and corn.

Now some suggestions, roughly in a time sequence, for plants, for both speciality and commodity crops:

- development of rapid genetic typing methods to speed conventional plant breeding, with the identification of genes responsible for desirable traits, and their transfer to other species; for example, between the cereals, which have been shown to have a common genetic map;

- development of plants resistant to many herbicides and a wide varity of pathogens, including viruses, bacteria and fungi, thus greatly reducing or eliminating the huge losses due to these agents;

- continued development of novel fertility systems, leading to the production of new F1 hybrids, with increased yields;

- continued development of fruits and vegetables with longer shelf lives and better shipping characteristics;

- modification of fatty acid synthetic pathways to produce novel starches and oils containing different and more suitable fats, for either dietary or industrial use;

- modification of fruits and vegetables to improve flavour, texture and nutritional content; elimination of genes for toxicants and allergens;

- isolation and utilization of more complex genetic systems such as those controlling salt tolerance and drought resistance, making possible the production of plants which can be grown in a much wider variety of habitats;

- isolation of the genes that control development means that we can start to manipulate flower shape and colour for the horticultural industry;

- similar isolation of the genes that control the plant's response to day length means that it may be possible, by modifying these genes, to produce plants that come to maturity more quickly, and so (in the Northern Hemisphere) push north, for example the northern limit for growth of rape in Canada;

- production of drugs and vaccines in plants.

Developments in animals are currently aimed, in a way that I will describe later, primarily at the production of high-value/low-volume drugs from transgenic animals. Other developments will be much slower; for public concerns are more serious. But some predictions are possible.

- Development of rapid genetic typing techniques will revolutionize animal breeding, enabling the identification of the genes critical for elite stocks and their transfer, by conventional breeding, to others, using cattle, pigs and horses or poultry.

- Similarly, the identification of genes for undesirable traits will accelerate our ability to remove them from breeding stock.

- Better understanding of infectious disease pathogens should lead to the ability to breed animals with increased disease resistance.

- Genes could be introduced to enable cows to produce milk that is much closer in its composition to human milk for feeding to babies.

- A similar approach could be used to produce transgenic animals with, for example, less body fat. However, it will, I think, be some time before such animals are acceptable for food.

Consumer Reactions

And what does the consumer think of all these changes? Let me tell you some issues that came to the Advisory Committee on Novel Foods and Processes, which I chaired for nine years, issues that helped us to learn about public attitudes. We used to think, we experts, that all we had to do was to decide whether a novel food or process was safe or not and a grateful public would accept what we said. That's not so, and we learnt our lessons the hard way; by getting something wrong. *Nothing is gained by even appearing to withhold information from the consumer.*

In late 1988, we were asked to approve the use of a genetically modified baker's yeast, developed by introducing two genes from a similar yeast, in order to increase the rate at which bread rose. This seemed to us a good case with which to start. After all, the genetic change could have been brought about by the naturally occurring yeast mating process. We could not see any problem and said so, and in early 1990 a brief press release appeared which announced that 'the product may be used safely'. The press, however, was distinctly unenthusiastic. Comments varied from: 'Genetic yeast passed for use' in *The Times*, through 'Man-made yeast raises temperature' in the *Independent*, to 'Bionic bread sales wrapped in secrecy' in *Today*, and 'Are the boffins taking the rise out of bread?' in the *Star*. The Consumers' Association said: 'We think all genetically altered foods should be labelled' – a reaction so negative that the product has never been used.

As a result of this, a consumer representative and an ethical advisor, John Polkinghorne, were added to our Committee. We also made the process much more transparent, producing annual reports and holding annual press conferences. Press releases were produced before and after each meeting of the ACNFP, as well as after Ministerial approval of each product or process, and I spent a good deal of time talking to journalists informally over the phone. *We learnt that decisions involving the public being exposed to any risk not of their own choosing must be taken as openly as possible.*

Then, about five years ago, we were asked whether meat from genetically modified sheep could enter the food chain. These sheep carried the human gene for Factor IX, a protein involved in blood clotting and needed for the treatment of haemophiliacs. The process involves injection of the purified gene into the fertilized sheep egg, before reimplantation and rearing. However, it sometimes takes over 100 animals to be reared before one animal is produced which can yield Factor IX in high quantities. We were asked whether the animals which either contained no novel genes, or an inactive novel gene, could be eaten. We could not think of any reason why animals without any foreign DNA should not be eaten. But were newspapers going to run the headline 'Failures from genetic engineering in your supermarket'? What about the animals containing an inactive human gene? Was this just a stretch of DNA like any other? Or was it special, because it came from a human being? Would eating sheep meat containing a single human gene even be regarded as cannibalism by some? Would Muslims or Jews be concerned about pork genes in lamb, and vegetarians about animals genes in plants? We did not know, but decided that it was probably a wider issue than one of pure technical safety, and suggested wider consultation to the Government.

This found that the Christians were divided. Many had an uneasy concern, a feeling shared by others, which has been termed the 'yuk' factor. The Jewish reaction was more straightforward: 'If it looks like a sheep, then it's a sheep' was their comment. Muslims and Hindus were much more opposed, as were the animal welfare groups, and also the vegetarians. Most groups were concerned, even if the gene was completely synthetic, and also because of the 'slippery slope' argument. These sheep had only one human gene in 100,000 sheep genes. But what if they had a 50:50 mixture of human and sheep genes? Then I think all of us would be concerned. People were worried too, about labelling, and wanted consumers to have choice. There was obviously quite widespread unease. The result is that even the animals with no foreign genes will not enter the food chain. *Consumer concerns, even if they do not appear to have a rational basis to scientists, must be taken seriously, and not brushed aside.*

A different issue surfaced over a herbicide-resistant soya, genetically modified by the introduction of a gene from a soil bacterium to make the soya resistant to the herbicide glyphosate. We had no safety concerns, and the Food Advisory Committee did not require labelling because it was substantially equivalent to the existing product. It did, however, recommend the provision of information on a voluntary basis by the retailer, the practice followed in the case of the successful launch of the paste from genetically modified tomatoes earlier in the year. Yet, with soya, as you may know, there has been substantial consumer concern because the retailers have not been able to offer their customers the choice between a modified and an unmodified product. This is because it has proved impossible to segregate the genetically modified soya from 'normal' soya at the source. Despite the best efforts of the retailers, who have provided a range of useful information leaflets and the provision of a helpline, there has been this consumer concern because of the absence of choice. *Consumers want to make their own, informed decisions.*

So, let me sum up the lessons we have learnt.

- Nothing is gained by even appearing to withhold information from the consumer.

- When decisions involve the public being exposed to any risk not of their own choosing, they must be taken as openly as possible.

- Consumer concerns, even if they do not appear to have a rational basis to scientists, must be taken seriously, and not brushed aside.

- Consumers want to make their own, informed decisions.

Why is this? Why do consumers want to make their own decisions? Basically, I think, because they have lost a lot of confidence in what they hear from politicians and, to a lesser extent, from regulators. And what are the reasons for this loss of consumer confidence? Let me suggest several.

- First, scientists, and the expert approval processes, are no longer trusted as they once were. The 'man in the white laboratory coat' no longer recommends washing powder – the consumer does. And public confidence in the regulatory process has been severely damaged by the BSE and *E. coli* outbreaks.

- Second, the public is largely unaware of the development of careful scientific methods of assessing risk, such as the use of hazard analysis to come much closer to an 'objective' evaluation of risk. But it is also true that we find great difficulty in explaining, and the public in understanding, what is meant by different degrees of risk. Our National Lottery – with its slogan of 'It could be you' – does not help either. The message is clear: even what is very unlikely may happen. It has been pointed out that you are more likely to die while watching the National Lottery than win the jackpot, but that does not stop people buying tickets; someone has to win! So even if the risk from a new product is very low, maybe it will be me!

- Third, the public finds it difficult to know how seriously to take the points put by the many single-issue pressure groups, such as Greenpeace and others.

- Fourth, risks are assessed differently according to the context. We will accept quite high risks when we are seriously ill, but will not tolerate much risk at all with food.

> Medicine is restoring natural function to an organism
> already threatened, but food is the 'staff of life', a basic
> good that must not be threatened.

One explanation for such conflicting views is that scientists and the public work from different value systems. Scientists and technologists see novel applications of new discoveries as logical and reasonable – and characterize all opposition as unreasonable. 'If only they understood what we are doing,' they say, 'the public would agree with us.' So there is much emphasis on what is called 'the public understanding of science', which I am sure is helpful, but it does always assume the scientist's value system as its starting point. Scientists are used to an uncertain world, where knowledge is always flawed. They can handle risk judgements more easily, and are impatient of those who cannot.

The public's reaction is quite different. It is more likely to be characterized by outrage – 'how dare they do this to us?'; dread – the way we would regard a nuclear power station explosion; and stigma – the way the public regard food irradiation. As a result, scientists are regarded as arrogant, distant and uncaring. That's not a good image for science or for scientists.

The roles of the scientist and the wider public have become confused too. Scientists and technologists used to make the decision about whether a new risk was acceptable to the public or not, in what now seems a rather a paternalistic fashion. Consumer groups now often make statements about the level of risk in an area where the science is very complex, and where simple conclusions are not easy to draw, for example in ecology. Surely, the assessment of risk is the responsibility of the scientist, while the wider community, and ultimately the politicians, must decide whether that risk is worth taking.

Playing God?

There is another concern expressed by the public, for some think that scientists are playing God. The public asks 'How do you know you are not going to release a new plague?' Scientists reply that they see living systems as a unity, knowing that cells, from bacteria to human beings, work in much the same way. So of course it is all right to move genes around – all we have to do is to explain it clearly, and people will be reassured. We are not abusing our position as the earth's most powerful species. We know what we are doing.

I think this is all too glib. There are, first of all, important technical issues to be talked about, particularly environmental issues. Will herbicide resistance spread to weeds, will antibiotic-resistant genes transfer from plants to humans through gut bacteria, will the use of the Bt gene in the potato, to provide protection against insect pests, also have a deleterious effect on the ladybird population, and so prevent their mopping up the aphids, as a recent report suggests? These environmental issues are regulated by the Advisory Committee on Release into the Environment (ACRE). It is being careful and cautious, insisting on a series of controlled trials; first in a contained greenhouse, then in a carefully isolated field plot, before finally going out to planting. The pollen dispersal and the adjacent flora are being monitored to see if there is any spread of the genetically modified (GM) crop. So far we are all right, but the situation needs careful watching, and concerns have been expressed that the 'case by case' approach used by the Committee will not deal with the sum of a series of decisions about release. It is therefore good news that an industry-wide code on GM-crop information has very recently been launched by the National Farmers' Union, which aims to ensure traceability and best practice in use by establishing a consistent approach to information-transfer for UK-grown crops from initial stock to primary end product. In addition, the Nuffield Council on Bioethics formed a Working Party which has recently produced a report on the Genetic Modification of Crops: The Social and Ethical Issues.

But there are other issues. There is the natural/unnatural issue. Some think that it is unwise, even unethical, to disturb the natural world – and that genetic modification is unnatural because it crosses species barriers. Others believe that BSE resulted from the 'unnatural', feeding of an animal foodstuff to a herbivore; in their view, BSE is a sort of divine judgement for upsetting the natural order of things. Now personally, I do not accept that all that is natural is best; fungal infection of crops with production of the ergot alkaloids is certainly not for the good of those who eat the crops. And why the yoghurt that I eat for my lunch is better for containing 'natural' colouring defeats me! Is there an issue here, or are we too romantic about what is 'natural'?

For the Christian, the fundamental question is whether any interference in 'the natural' or created order is permitted or not. If so, what criteria are to be used in establishing the limits of such inteference? Biblical teaching sees human beings with the responsibility of stewardship for all creation, but this has not excluded us intervening in the natural world, ever since we ceased to be hunter-gatherers. The question, then, is whether the genetic constitution of living creatures, a constitution that has undoubtedly changed during the course of evolution, should have any specially protected status. That is, is it wrong *in principle*? I do not think so, though that is not to say that individual cases might not be unwise or even wicked, and should not proceed.

But to go back to the beginning: why were the people we consulted so resistant to the idea of eating a human gene? Even when it was totally synthetic? Partly, I think, because they do not know where to draw the line between one gene and a thousand. Is this the start of a slippery slope? However, we must surely be able to draw a line somewhere? We aleady do so in other cases, for example in the case of experiments on very early human embryos.

But I think there is another reason as well. I suspect that people think that there is something special about human genes. Is there a concern about what science is doing to our perception of humanness? People are loving, caring, choosing human beings, with deeply held beliefs and values, many of which are central to their view of what a human being is. They accept the centrality of our genes – but not that we are no more than a bunch of genes. So they think that there must be something special about human genes, which must not be treated merely as chemicals. Is this a reaction to reductionism? A rejection of the idea that we are nothing but a bunch of genes? The concern of the public is not lessened by the aggressive determinism of some current biologists, or the slant of some of the science-education initiatives. Calling man 'the third chimpanzee' does not help.

Let me try and sort out some of these different ethical issues and see how our Christian faith can help us. First, there is a clear warning to us scientists who are Christians, that in stressing the underlying simplicity and order of the complex world which modern biology reveals, and in stressing the power and effectiveness of modern technology, we must also stress its limits. We must be less assertive, less arrogant than is sometimes the case at present. We are too often driven by our love of new technology, and are unaware of the dehumanizing effect of the innate reductionism that is the basis of modern molecular biology. So we are regarded as arrogant, distant and uncaring. That is a warning to us all.

Second, we scientists working in the food area must be sensitive to the different way in which the general public regards new technology when it is applied to food. Let me digress for a moment. In both Greek and Latin, ethics and morals originally meant simply 'custom' or 'habit' – and we still have this meaning in English in the words 'ethos' and 'mores'. Despite these origins, 'ethics' and 'morality' now usually entail 'values' and 'principles' which most people believe should not be reduced simply to 'customs' and 'habits'. In our area of novel foods and processes both sets of meanings are involved. Food is surrounded by 'customs' and 'habits' which can properly change over time. Some of these customs derive from religious traditions (e.g. Jews and Muslims not eating pork) and others probably have secular origins (e.g. the English not eating dogs or horses). Breaking these customs can be very offensive to other people but it is not clear that they actually involve wrongdoing as such. They are, perhaps, much more to do with social and community identity, which of course is becoming weaker in our increasingly pluralistic world. However, other aspects of novel foods and processes are much more to do with values, especially the fundamental value of not harming the innocent. So allowing novel foods which risk harm to the innocent would be wrong. It is therefore a clear moral/ethical duty for those developing novel foods and processes to test their safety extremely carefully, and it may always be right to err on the side of caution when there might be risk. It is also necessary to be sensitive to the difference between the consumer's attitude to change in medicine and food; the practices are not simply transferable.

Third, there is the natural/unnatural issue that I raised earlier, and I think that there are a number of issues here.

First, although this is a distinction commonly made by non-scientists, it is a distinction that all scientists, including Christians, find difficult to understand. We who are Christians see no distinction between what we learn of the world through our faith and through our science; what we do in the laboratory is not 'unnatural'. It is all God's world.

Second, this distinction assumes a false, I believe, romantic view of 'Nature', a view verging on pantheism. The world is not ideally left as it is; rivers do need taming, land use has to change if we are to feed our world, and all environments need managing. This view assumes that much modern agriculture is 'unnatural', but I have an uneasy feeling that some of these concerns are only possible for us because we are so affluent and can afford to pay more, as we surely will, for (say) non-genetically modified soya – although the genetically modified form is a product which I believe carries no health risk. So if customers want to choose, then they will have to pay. That is not an option for many in the developing world, for they need the food.

Third, though it is impossible to distinguish between 'natural' vanilla and that made by chemistry or fermentation, some want to buy 'natural' vanilla because by doing so they are maintaining a Third World economy. But that is not a problem peculiar to biotechnology. Every time we replace an imported raw material by one derived from high technology (and there are many reasons or doing so) we are into this debate, which is much more complex than it sounds, and which too easily tempts well-intentioned but uninformed people into pronouncements about economics.

Fourth, there are environmental issues. It was Edmund Burke who said: 'Society is indeed a contract [. . .] it becomes a partnership between not only those who are living, but between those who are living, those who are dead, and those who are yet to be born.' This seems to me to be a deeply biblical idea. Have we got our present practices right? I am beginning to get concerned that we are being insufficiently careful as to our responsibility to future generations. We have to be very careful.

Finally, there is the lack of moral acceptability of some theoretical outcomes of genetic engineering, sometimes called the 'yuk' factor, which might be exemplified by considering why some would not wish to eat an animal that contained even a single human gene in 100,000 sheep genes. If that might be acceptable, would an animal with 10 or 100 or 1,000 human genes be acceptable? We can draw the line somewhere, and why? Is it something to do with the integrity of the individual – using people as things? And is this the 'bridge too far'? Certainly a recent Europe-wide survey published in *Nature* (Vol. 387, 26 June 1997, pp. 845–7), which found that 'risk is less significant than moral acceptability in shaping public perceptions of biotechnology', shows how important understanding what lies behind our concerns is. How can we define the issues, and a public policy that deals with them?

So, to sum up: I believe this new technology has the capacity to make food cheaper, safer and more nutritious. There are few quantifiable risks to the consumer, but their concerns, which are much more about moral acceptability, need to be handled thoughtfully and openly. We do not have the right to use a new technology unless the users or consumers, or at least most of them, are happy about it. That means open dialogue, and when in doubt, delay. With those provisos, we can thank God for another insight into this amazing world we live in, and our ability to use our knowledge for the good of all.

Suggested Reading

M.J. Reiss and R. Straughan, *Improving Nature? The Science and Ethics of Genetic Engineering.* Cambridge, Cambridge University Press, 1996.

G. Conway, *The Doubly Green Revolution: Food for All in the 21st Century.* London, Penguin, 1997.

CHAPTER FOUR

Transplantation Ethics: What it Means to be Human

Michael Rees

In the last chapter, Derek Burke asked whether it was right to eat the meat of sheep that had undergone a genetic manipulation intended to give the sheep a human gene. As he pointed out, only about 1 in 100 of the sheep so manipulated actually get the gene into the right place. His committee was asked if it was acceptable for the public to eat the 99 sheep out of 100 that underwent the manipulation, but did not appear to have the gene transferred to them. He wondered whether we might be considered cannibals if we ate lamb meat that had a human gene in it. What he was really asking was whether or not it is our DNA that makes us human. Is isolated human DNA special and protectable in the same way that you or I are special and protectable? Is each person's DNA what makes them special? Is an isolated piece of human DNA to be regarded as special compared to a piece of mouse DNA, just as a human life is special compared with a mouse life?

Derek Burke went on to suggest an amusing answer to these questions. He wondered whether we are being cannibals when we nibble on our fingernails and digest the human DNA contained within them. I certainly hope not! What if it was not my fingernail I nibbled on and digested, but yours? Would that be cannibalism? Obviously the answer there is a humorous 'no'. What about blood transfusion or organ donation where the DNA of another human actually becomes a part of us? Is this practice equivalent to cannibalism? And if not, does that mean that it is not our DNA or our organs that make us human? If our DNA or our individual organs are not what make us human, what does? These are the issues I want to discuss in this chapter, and I hope to challenge you to reconsider what it means to be human, to be different from animals in a way that is more than just physical; perhaps to see us as human and alive from the vantage point of God.

I do not want to discuss whether we humans are more valuable than animals, or whether there is a God; I admit up front that I take those things for granted. So, if you are an atheist, or a naturalist who believes that all living creatures share equal value, or think that there are no ultimate rights and wrongs in the universe, then you will disagree with my starting premises. But if you think there might be a God, or that in some undefined way human life is more valuable than the lives of other creatures in our world, then I hope to challenge you to define what it means to be human, by helping you to understand better what it means not to be human.

Imagine that you are a transplant surgeon. It is 3 o'clock in the morning and the phone is ringing. You answer it, and hear the voice of your transplant co-ordinator informing you that someone in a city two hours away has been declared brain-dead and their family has given permission for your transplant team to harvest the organs from their deceased loved one. You ask the relevant questions, ingrained from years of training, which allow you to determine if the potential organ donor is an appropriate candidate from a medical perspective. A few moments later, you give the go ahead for the co-ordinator to organize the team that will change the lives of several patients with end-stage organ failure. As you shower and dress for the long day ahead, you hope that, in some small way, the efforts you exert in the next few hours will ease the pain of the family who has just suffered a tragic loss.

And the losses are always tragic. A three-year-old boy who died of meningitis; an 18-year-old girl killed by a drunk driver; a 52-year-old woman expecting her first grandchild next week who collapsed at home from a cerebral haemorrhage. But just as the losses are tragic, so the transplant recipient stories are joyful. A three-year-old boy, the only child of doting parents, is given a new heart and a new lease on life; an 18-year-old girl struck down with a rare liver disease is saved from the brink of death; finally, a 52-year-old woman whom kidney transplantation frees from the chains of dialysis so that she can travel halfway around the world to see the birth of her first grandchild.

While there is no doubt that transplantation is a clinical reality today because of several medical breakthroughs, in this chapter we are discussing the philosophical and ethical assumptions behind transplantation. After that, I will take you on a journey into the future to explore potential new ways of replacing human organs.

Death

Prior to the seventeenth century people were considered to be dead when they stopped breathing. In 1628 William Harvey discovered that the heart pumped blood around the body, and our understanding of being dead changed to the concept of being dead when the heart stopped. The advent of cardiopulmonary bypass and heart surgery in the 1960s changed our perception of death again. No longer could we think of being dead as when the heart stopped, because clearly people whose hearts were stopped during a heart operation were not dead. This difficulty left us without a definitive way of describing death. By the 1970s, we could rescue someone outside the hospital by starting CPR (cardiopulmonary resuscitation), rushing them to the hospital, and immediately using a respirator to breathe for them. By so doing, doctors often found themselves in the position of ventilating someone whose brain was dead and thus had no chance of long-term survival. But by using artificial breathing, the doctors could keep the rest of the body alive for an indefinite period of time. This raised both ethical and economic concerns. It is very expensive to keep someone alive in an intensive care unit and health-care resources are limited. The grieving family was forced to linger, waiting for the rest of the body to join the brain in death. These considerations forced doctors to re-evaluate the definition of death and we decided that when your brain was dead, you were dead.

But defining death is not such an easy thing. Did you know that when you die, the actual tissues of your body die at different rates? For instance, I could take a biopsy of the muscles of your leg several hours after you were dead and cold and I could find live muscle cells. I could even get them to grow in a dish in a laboratory and make new cells. It is possible that a part of you could go on living in that sense for years after you were dead. There are reports of facial hair in dead people growing for days after death. So, death has to be thought of as a process rather than a precise event. The question is what body part or function has to be permanently lost before we consider someone to be dead.

What do you think defines being alive? Clearly it is not the loss of the ability to breathe, as there are thousands of people on breathing machines at this moment around the world. Nor is it the loss of the heart, as we routinely replace failed hearts, and the patient is not regarded as dead when they are without a heart. Equally, a person who has a few cells in his big toe alive while the rest of his body is dead is regarded as dead long before reaching that point. The difficult question that we face as a society today is to decide when in the process of dying someone passes over the boundary of being alive to being dead. As I will show, this is important, not only for helping a grieving family, and for allocating precious health-care resources, but in making transplantation the clinical reality it is today.

Once someone has died, the organs and cells of their body begin the irreversible process of dying which ends when the last cell of the body dies. The organs and cells of the body die at different rates after death. Without oxygen, the organs of the body are the first to lose the ability to function, though individual cells within the organ may still be alive even though the organ itself is considered to be dead. Also, different organs lose the ability to function at different rates after death. For instance, brain tissue dies within minutes if it does not receive oxygen, followed by the heart, and then the liver, and then the kidneys. This is best illustrated by how quickly we have to transplant a particular organ once it has been removed from the body. A heart preserved with special fluid and packed on ice can only survive up to four hours, a liver up to 8 to 12 hours, while kidneys can last 24 to 48 hours. Without the special preservation fluid and being packed in ice, these times are significantly shorter, so that human organs left in a warm body without circulating blood die within the first hour after the patient has died. So, just as I could find living cells in a dead organ, I could find living organs in a dead person. It is this concept that allows people to make a gift of their organs upon their death.

Brainstem Death

By defining someone as being dead when their brain has died, modern medicine can place us in a situation where a person is dead but some of their organs are still alive. They are alive, because doctors have used artificial means of life support to keep that person's organs alive. For example, Mr Jones has epilepsy and one day he has a seizure five minutes before his wife gets home. After his seizure he stops breathing, but his heart continues to beat. Several minutes after Mr Jones' seizure, his brain is dead from lack of oxygen, but his other organs are still alive. At this moment, his wife, who is a nurse, comes through the door and begins to administer CPR. Minutes later an ambulance crew arrives and Mr Jones is brought to the local emergency room. A breathing tube is inserted into his lungs and a breathing machine performs the one function your body cannot do without a brain – namely breathe. (Your heart can keep beating without a brain, but you need your brain to breathe.) In the days before all of our fancy medical technology, we could not separate the functions of the body in this way. If your heart stopped, your brain soon died; or if your brain died, you stopped breathing and soon your heart stopped. Now we find ourselves being able to replace the function of various organs of the body with machines, and these machines sometimes bring us to a situation where Mr Jones has a dead brain but living organs. Is Mr Jones dead?

Legally, Mr Jones is considered to be dead if his brain is dead, regardless of the state of the rest of his body. Do you agree with this concept of death? And, those of you who believe in the concept of a soul, if you are brain dead, does your soul do whatever one's soul does when one dies? I have thought a great deal about this question and for good reason. In order to transplant organs from dead people into living people, I have to remove living organs from someone who is dead, so that these organs can remain living in the new recipient of the transplant.

Let me illustrate this point more graphically. Assume that Mr Jones generously made it known during his lifetime that he wanted to be an organ donor upon his death, and that his family consented to this wish. The body of Mr Jones would then be taken to the operating room with his heart still beating, the breathing machine still providing oxygen to his blood, and his internal organs still alive. As the surgeon operating on him, I would make an incision from his chest to the lower part of his abdomen and operate for several hours to prepare the organs for removal. When everything was ready we would then infuse cold fluid specially designed to preserve the organs, and I would cut the big blood vessel that connects the lower half of the body to the heart. In so doing, Mr Jones' blood would empty into his chest. If he was not already dead when he was brought to the operating room, he would be now. I think about that every time I cut that big blood vessel. I clearly have made the decision that Mr Jones was dead the moment his brain died. I hope that God and those who look back on our current practice of transplantation hundreds or thousands of years from now also view a patient, defined as dead by today's brain-death criteria, as really being dead. I cannot imagine it otherwise. But I do not believe William Harvey in 1628 imagined that I could hold his heart in my hand and he could still be alive.

In Search of Organs

While much more could be said about our concepts of brain death, death describes only one aspect of human life – the end. Understanding better what it means to be dead is only just the beginning of our exploration of what it means to be human. In fact, I think the question of brain death is the easiest of the questions I will raise in this chapter. Let us now look into the question of what it means to be human by asking how far we can go in our search for organs to transplant into humans.

Because of the success of organ transplantation, today we face a chronic shortage of donor organs. It is estimated that in America alone 100,000 people a year could be treated with heart transplantation. As there are only 10,000 organ donors per year, that leaves 90,000 people a year dying who could be saved if additional hearts were available for transplantation. The situation is similar for other organs we commonly transplant such as kidneys, livers and pancreases.

One of the new approaches which is being investigated is the possibility of using animals as a source of organs for transplantation. You may have heard of previous attempts to use chimpanzee, baboon or pig organs for transplantation into humans. Until recently, the transplantation of organs from one species into another has been impossible because of a severe immune response, which rejects the animal organ within minutes of stitching it into place. Recent discoveries have improved our understanding in this area and it now appears possible that, by genetic engineering, we may be able to use animal organs for transplantation into humans. This is fraught with ethical questions such as whether it is right to use animals in this way, or whether animal organs might transmit horrible viruses that otherwise could not infect us. But those are not the focus of this chapter. Let us again assume that a human life is more valuable than an animal's life so that, from an ethical point of view, using an animal's organs for transplantation is no worse than eating the meat of an animal. What I want to consider are the means that are being employed to try to use animal organs in transplantation.

Is DNA What Makes Us Human?

As Derek Burke described, plants and animals are routinely being genetically engineered. This is the approach that is being used to try to produce animals whose organs could be transplanted into humans. It turns out that we humans have specialized proteins on the surface of our cells that protect us from our own immune system. You can think of it as like a protective shield. When our immune system tries to destroy something that has invaded us like a bacterium or virus, our immune system attacks it just as our military would attack an invading country's forces. But in war, you want to destroy only military targets and to avoid injuring civilian targets. The military call this 'minimizing collateral damage'. The same concept applies when your immune system attempts to destroy something. It aims specifically to bomb the bad things that have invaded your body, while avoiding injury to your own tissues.

But, as in the conflict in Kosovo, no matter how sophisticated the laser-guided bombs are, they sometimes miss their target and bomb something they were not intended to destroy. The same thing goes on inside our body all the time. Most of the time we destroy whatever bad thing we are aiming at inside our body, but occasionally our immune system misses and bombs us. Fortunately, we have a protective coating that keeps the immune bombs of our body from destroying our own cells. Now, all animals have a similar coating; monkeys have monkey-protective coatings, pigs have pig-protective coatings and so on. The question is: will a pig-protective coating protect a pig cell from human immune bombs? The answer turns out to be no. So, the reason that organs from one species get rejected so quickly when they are transplanted into the body of another species is that the cells of one species cannot protect themselves from the immune system of another species.

So, how could we protect the cells of a pig, for instance, from a human immune system? We could genetically engineer the pig so that it had the human protective shield on the surface of all of its cells. How does one do that? You take the fertilized egg of a pig and you hold it on the end of a very small glass tube, as though you were sucking on it through a straw. Then, once you have the fertilized egg in position, you take a very small needle and stick it into the middle of the cell, into the nucleus. You then inject a million copies of the human gene that codes for the human protective shield and hope that one of those millions of copies of the same gene somehow inserts itself into one of the chromosomes of the pig. You then take the injected fertilized pig egg and put it into the uterus of a pig. When the piglets are born, you check them to see if the human gene is inserted somewhere into one of the pig chromosomes. This does not happen very frequently, so that perhaps only 1 out of 100 of the newborn pigs will have the human gene for the human protective shield. But, because all the cells of the pig came from the one fertilized egg, every cell of the pig where the human gene somehow got in will have that gene. And because every cell has that gene, every pig cell will now have a human protective shield. You can also use that 1 out of 100 pigs to breed new pigs that will have the human gene, because the human gene will be carried in all of the sperm or eggs of such genetically engineered pigs.

My second question is: is this activity acceptable? Is it appropriate for human beings to make an animal that has one human gene in it? Does that diminish the value of a human being? Is the pig so engineered so much like a human that it is no longer a pig, but some kind of pig/human hybrid, to be treated with more reverence than a normal pig but perhaps not as much reverence as a human? If putting one human gene into a pig is all right, are two genes all right? Or ten? Or 100? Can you imagine a situation where you could put all of the human genetic material into a pig cell and still regard that as acceptable?

Cloning and Beyond

Let us assume that after giving this some thought, you decide that a few human genes are acceptable but you do not want to go too far down the slippery slope. You might argue that putting too many human genes into a pig cell would make it a human rather than a pig – and that would be wrong. Before reaching too firm a conclusion, however, allow me to take you on a journey into the world of science fiction. The things I am going to describe now are not yet being done, but let us assume they are possible. I do not want to discuss whether such things are possible but whether, if they were possible, we should pursue them.

Let me set the stage by reminding you of what John Polkinghorne said about how Dolly the sheep was cloned. The scientists took an unfertilized egg from a black sheep, stuck a needle into the egg, and sucked out all of the genetic material contained within the nucleus. They then scraped the udder of a white sheep, took one of the mature mammary cells, and put that next to the black sheep unfertilized egg with no nucleus. They zapped these two cells with a bit of electricity, and the two cells fused and became one. Then an amazing thing happened: the new cell began to divide. They took the resulting clump of cells and placed it into the uterus of a black sheep. A few months later, a white sheep had been born, genetically identical to the white sheep from which the udder cell had been obtained.

Until January of 1998, scientists believed that mature cells could not go backwards to become less mature cells. We thought that cells could only go in the direction of being more differentiated, not less differentiated so that only egg and sperm cells, or early foetal cells, had the ability to grow into all the parts of a body. But cloning has changed all that. Somehow, the stuff in a cell outside the nucleus can influence the nucleus so that it can go backwards in time, and recover the ability to make all the various parts of a body.

Do Organs Make Us Human?

Let us consider a slight modification of this process. Imagine that we have the capability to operate on a little pig embryo no bigger than a millimetre or two. Imagine also that we can identify which cells are destined to become the pig kidney and remove them when there are only four or so of them. Now, suppose that you need a new kidney. You go to your local transplant centre and they take a sample of your blood. They take one of your white blood cells and they put it next to one of these early kidney cells of a pig embryo from which the nucleus has been removed. They zap it with electricity, and soon it fuses into one cell and begins to divide. When it reaches the four-cell stage they get another pig embryo, operate on it and remove the four cells on one side that were going to be one of that pig's kidneys. They then replace those four pig cells with the four cells resulting from the fusion of your cell and another pig's early kidney cells. Finally, they close up the pig embryo and put it back into its mother. When that piglet is born, it has a pig kidney on one side and your kidney on the other. Because pigs grow much faster than humans, within six months the pig has grown to be the same size as you, and the kidney has become the proper size for transplantation. So, within a year of your being diagnosed with kidney failure, a new organ has been specially designed for you that can be transplanted, without all of the immunosuppressive drugs and risks currently required in transplantation.

Would such an action be acceptable? Would it be appropriate to put our entire human DNA into a pig cell? Would such a pig be more like a human, some kind of pig/human hybrid, to be treated with more reverence than a normal pig but perhaps not as much reverence as a human? Let us say that you need a heart, and another needs a liver, and a third needs a kidney. Would it be all right to grow a pig with a human heart, liver, kidney and pancreas as long as on the outside it still looked like a pig? What if the human part we needed to replace was visible on the outside of the pig? Would that make it less acceptable? Perhaps you had lost your arm in an accident and the only way to grow a new one was to grow it on a pig. Would a pig with human arms be acceptable? If not, and yet you agreed with growing a human kidney hidden within the pig, what is the philosophical principle that justifies using a pig to grow a human kidney, but not to grow a human arm? If you do agree with growing these human parts, where do you draw the line? What if you gave the pig a human brain? One could then certainly argue that you had crossed the line.

What is it that defines a pig as a pig, and a human as a human? Let us assume, difficult though some of these ideas are on first hearing them, that you decide on further reflection that as long as they are applied in the noble cause of saving someone's life, they are justifiable. What you will then have conceded is the following. When someone is brain dead, they are dead and their soul has done what souls do when we die. Human DNA is not what makes us human, as part or all of it can be manipulated for a good cause. Human organs are not of themselves what defines us as humans, and they can be manipulated for a good cause. The human brain, however, seems to be the exception. It is the organ that defines what makes us both human and alive. But what is it about the brain that separates us from animals? Is it our self-awareness, our ability to choose right from wrong, our capacity for intellect? Perhaps we are struggling to define that special something because it is not something that science can define. Perhaps we struggle because what makes us human and set apart from animals is not our brain or our mind, but our spirit. And whatever clever things we humans get up to, we will never genetically engineer the soul. St Matthew reminds us not to be afraid of those who kill the body but cannot kill the soul. 'Rather, be afraid of the One who can destroy both soul and body in hell' (Matthew 10.28 NIV).

Babies without Brains

Let me come now to what I believe is the most challenging of the possibilities I want to consider, and perhaps the one that we are closest to making a reality. Again, it is but science fiction today, but if we could do it, should we?

Let us return to the concept of cloning. Again, let us say that you need a kidney. We draw your blood. We take an unfertilized pig egg, remove the nucleus and put your white blood cell next to the empty unfertilized pig egg. We shock it with electricity and wait for the fusion. After the cell begins to divide, we do not put it into a pig

45

to grow up, but rather grow millions and millions of copies of that cell in a laboratory dish. You will recall that I told you that it is rare to get a little piece of DNA into the chromosome of a cell. There are other genetic modifications that are even rarer, so rare that to try it one at a time, as in injecting a fertilized egg, would be futile. But if you treated ten million cells all at once, you could select the one in ten million genetic event. So, by having ten million identical copies of a cell that has your DNA, it is possible to alter one of your pre-existing genes, not just randomly add a new gene. For the purpose of this discussion, let us say that the gene we alter is the gene that controls the formation of the brain. Out of the ten million cells in the laboratory dish, we select the one cell in which this gene has been destroyed and we transfer it into a pig uterus. Several months later, what has grown inside that pig uterus is you as you were as a newborn infant, but without a brain. The medical term is an anencephalic infant.

Anencephaly takes many forms, from missing most of the brain to missing all of the brain. So, a child could be born with only a brainstem and none of the rest of the brain. Such a child could breathe upon birth and by our current definitions of brain death would not be dead, though having no capacity for cognition. For the purpose of this discussion, let us assume that the anencephalic human produced never developed any part of the brain or brainstem. Such an infant would die immediately upon birth because, without a brainstem, it could not breathe.

But perhaps it is inaccurate to state that such an infant could die. One could argue that the infant was never alive – and therefore could not die, because it never had a brain or a brainstem. The organs of the anencephalic infant were kept alive *in utero* because the placenta acted like the artificial breathing machine and source of nutrition, just as we can replace these functions in brain-dead people in intensive care units today. Since the anencephalic infant is already dead, we could justify removing the kidneys and transplanting them into you. So we have purposefully produced an anencephalic clone of you for the express purpose of growing you a new kidney. If we could grow your kidney in an isolated laboratory dish we would, but we cannot. We require the almost magical embryological process to grow a kidney from scratch, and this can only take place inside a developing body in a uterus.

So is this acceptable? Can we morally, ethically, or philosophically justify designing anencephalic humans as an organ culture for patients with organ failure? Is an anencephalic infant any different from a brain-dead patient? If you have assented to the other ideas I have presented in this chapter, but this last idea is unacceptable, how do you justify your position? If you agree that brain death means that you are dead, that DNA is not what defines us as human and that organs are interchangeable from the neck down, what is it about anencephalic donors that you find so disturbing?

Some have described it as the 'yuk' factor. But is the 'yuk' factor a morally defensible basis for not doing something? When I cut open the soft delicate skin of a beautiful three-year-old girl who had died to take out her organs, I am filled with an overwhelming sense of 'yuk'. But I carry on because I believe what I am doing is a good thing, and will benefit my fellow man. Sometimes we have to do things that are 'yukky', not because we want to, but because it is the right thing to do. I wonder which of the ideas I have put before you in this chapter fall into this category.

Truth

The last paragraph might have been a good place to end this chapter. I developed the dilemma, pushed each technology to the extreme, and left you to decide what was right and wrong. But in many conversations regarding these topics, I find people responding that you just should not do one or the other of these things because it is disgusting, or they did not feel it was right, or it did not coincide with their belief system. Perhaps the most important question I have to ask you is this: Can we force our beliefs regarding the morality of a certain action on to a group of people with a different value system. And if we can, why?

Let us take the issue of animal rights. Suppose you believe that animals are just as special (or perhaps just as unspecial) as human beings and therefore we humans have no right to experiment on them, eat them, or use their body parts in any way for our benefit. Another person disgrees with you on each point and plans to eat beef, wear leather shoes, and humanely use animals in his research. According to our current post-modern world view, truth is whatever you think truth is, but we cannot really argue that my truth is any more valid than your truth. The alternative is that there is an ultimate truth with which we can judge the morality of any given situation. In this case, truth is not relative to individual human preference, but transcends and guides us.

The 'yuk' factor brings up perhaps the most important question of this chapter. For in a society where truth is relative and personal preference has replaced Truth, there are no rights and wrongs. When assessing whether a new technology is ethically acceptable, do we really want to base these decisions on what people can stomach, or is there a deeper basis for making them? Are there absolute truths we can base such decisions on or is absolute truth a myth?

I believe that God has revealed his truth to us in the Christian message. This is where I suggest we turn to find the answers to these difficult questions. I do not believe the answers are to be found in our present post-modern world view which suggests that truth is relative. For if truth is relative, then what is right is what society will tolerate. And is that how you think we should answer these questions – by gauging society's 'yuk factor'?

I hope this chapter has pushed you to the point that you have thought: 'NO, we cannot do such things – THAT IS WRONG!' And if I have pushed you to that point, is it wrong because of how you feel about it, or how I feel about it, or how society feels about it? Or, is it wrong because there is an absolute truth that speaks about what it means to be human and alive and specially set apart from other living creatures? I hope I have caused you to consider that it is not just our DNA or our organs that define us as human – but that it is our soul. And once we start our search for human worth with the soul, I believe it is much more likely that absolute truth will guide us in these difficult situations.

Suggested Reading

Further reading on the topic of brain death can be found in:

C.A. Pallis and D.H. Harley, *ABC of Brainstem Death*, 2nd edn. London, British Medical Journal Publishing Group, 1996.

A fascinating and disturbing book that explores issues of what it means to be human in terms of fertilization, cloning, embryos and DNA is:

L.M. Silver, *Remaking Eden: Cloning and Beyond in a Brave New World*. London, Weidenfeld & Nicolson, 1998.

Finally, Donald M. MacKay, a famous Scottish brain-researcher, gives an interesting twist to the relationship between brain, mind, body and soul in:

The Clockwork Image. Leicester, Inter-Varsity Press, 1974/1997.

The Open Mind and Other Essays. Leicester, Inter-Varsity Press, 1988.

CHAPTER FIVE

Reproductive Medicine

Tim Appleton

There have been many developments in reproductive medicine over the last forty years resulting in legislation and controls. Many people feel that the ability to manipulate the human embryo in the laboratory has meant that we are able to influence directly the quality of life at its very early stages – taking us beyond what nature had intended. In this chapter, I will restrict myself to the very beginning of the life, and look at some of the directions which assisted reproductive medicine is taking us in assisting childless couples where nature on its own has failed them.

On 25 July 1978 Patrick Steptoe delivered a baby to a woman with no fallopian tubes. He and his colleague Robert Edwards had successfully fertilized an egg in the laboratory and then transferred the embryo to the uterus of the mother.

Childlessness – Is it really a Disease?

Before the advent of the new reproductive technologies, which began with the birth of the first IVF baby, childlessness was something that many people had to accept and come to terms with. There was, after all, very little they could do about it other than to seek to adopt a child, an option which is strictly limited today – about 700 babies were available for adoption in England and Wales last year.

Today we have the ability:

- to take sperm and eggs and put them together in the laboratory;
- to create embryos in large numbers with comparative ease;

- to achieve pregnancies in women of any age by egg donation;
- to inject a single sperm directly into the embryo;
- to freeze excess embryos;
- to transfer embryos, eggs or sperms into surrogate mothers;
- to sex an early embryo or diagnose certain genetic abnormalities in a few cells taken from an eight-cell embryo by DNA amplification.

The fact that the technology exists makes it that much more difficult for many to come to terms with infertility. If the technology is there people want it, almost to the point of demanding it of right. Infertility becomes even harder to bear and leads to a sense of inadequacy, shame and anger, putting great strains on partnerships, marriages, family/friend relationships, and perhaps too on existing children from previous relationships. There is a sense of bereavement that begins from the moment that the problem is diagnosed. Many people are bruised by the inability of a State funded Health Service to cater for *all* the needs of *all* the people. Few couples will be offered free treatment, which they see *is* available in many other countries.

Many people will ask the question 'Is infertility really a disease?' After all, it is not life threatening. But what do we mean by the word 'disease' and where do we start to unravel the complexities of something we call infertility?

If we look in the Shorter Oxford Dictionary we find that the usage of the word 'disease' has at one period or another included 'absence of ease'; 'uneasiness'; 'inconvenience'; 'annoyance'; 'disturbance'; 'cause of discomfort'; 'a condition of the body or some part or organ of the body in which its functions are disturbed or deranged'; and 'diseased' means 'brought into a morbid or unhealthy state'.

We can certainly see all of those effects in those who suffer from infertility and so can describe infertility as a health-care problem *that should be tackled*. Those of us who have been fortunate in having children know the joys of having a family – even if we also experience the anguish that that also brings. Few of us would seriously expect to be permanently free of all the difficulties that go with parenthood.

Those who experience infertility feel helpless, having tried for so long without any signs of success. They are left out of a vital part of society – the family. Many may well have delayed having children until the job or house situation is more secure only to find that a problem in their fertility has either been there all along, or has progressively worsened over the years. These are, after all, often considered as taboo subjects that we do not easily share with others, and many find it difficult to talk about such sensitive matters as periods, menstrual cycles, sperm, eggs and so on.

The Church, I believe, has a positive role to play, since one of its prime concerns should be to be alongside the people within its pastoral care. In the past some sections of the Church have presented a rigid and negative face to infertility. We fear the unknown, and in that ignorance we conjure up possibilities for abuse which are already under careful control. There will always be areas that some will find disturbing while others can accept more pragmatically.

Abram and Sarai

We can see the effects of infertility in the biblical story of Abraham (Abram) and Sarah (Sarai) in Genesis 16.1–15; 17.15–19; 21.1–4; 25.12–18. It is an intriguing domestic triangle in which Sarah and Abraham seek with some impatience to provide the promised heir. William Neil in his *One Volume Bible Commentary* (Hodder & Stoughton, 1962) suggests that the compiler of the Book of Genesis had a perfectly adequate reason for including this story:

> The Bible consistently teaches us that God does not work according to man-made laws. It would almost seem as if one of the main messages of the Bible is to convince us that it is precisely what we should not expect that God does, precisely the people we should not choose that God chooses, precisely the moment that we should not judge appropriate God acts.

We can see with hindsight some of the problems that the initial solution to their problems brought and this emphasizes that we can never predict how events will turn out.

'Now Sarai, Abram's wife, bore him no children' (Genesis 16.1).

For Sarai the situation seemed quite simple. She says to Abram, 'The LORD has prevented me from bearing children; go in to my maid; it may be that I shall obtain children by her' (16.2). As a result of this relationship Hagar does conceive just as Sarah had intended. And this is just the start of a tortuous series of events which, while ending in happiness, is not without its difficulties. It was then, and still is, a radical way to solve the problem of childlessness. Yet it would be considered as a normal procedure in some African cultures – and certainly an accepted part of the wider family commitment.

Today surrogacy is considered as an ethical and emotional minefield that many would feel was an unacceptable solution to childlessness. Others would consider it as a 'last resort' solution acceptable in limited circumstances.

The account in Genesis does highlight some of the dangers which surrogacy brings.

- Hagar looked with contempt on her mistress (16.4).

- Sarai said to Abram, 'May the wrong done to me be on you! [...] When she [Hagar] saw that she had conceived, she looked on me with contempt' (16.5).

- The slave girl Hagar flees (16.6).

- Later on Hagar is found by 'the angel of the LORD' near a spring in the wilderness and told to return to her mistress, but his words contain both good news and bad: 'You ... shall bear a son ... He shall be a wild ass of a man, his hand against every man and every man's hand against him; and he shall dwell over against all his kinsmen' (16.11–12 RSV).

Hagar does indeed return and duly bears Abram a son, Ishmael, but now there are the questions of descent and identity. In establishing a covenant between God, Abraham and his descendants, questions are now raised about the place of Ishmael. Ishmael cannot be considered as a true descendant. 'O that Ishmael might live in thy sight!' Abraham says to God. But God replies, 'No, but Sarah your wife shall bear you a son, and you shall call his name Isaac. I will establish my covenant *with him* as an everlasting covenant for his descendants after him' (17.18–19). As for Ishmael, he has to be satisfied with a blessing and the promise to 'multiply him exceedingly' and that he will father twelve princes.

Sarah did conceive and bore Abraham a son (21.2). But the account does not end there, because later on Sarah sees Ishmael playing with her son Isaac (21.9) and is clearly angry because she too does not recognize Ishmael as her son. 'So she said to Abraham, "Cast out this slave woman with her son; for the son of this slave woman shall not be heir with my son Isaac"' (21.10). Although Abraham is clearly upset, he does as Sarah wants and God repeats his pledge to look after the lad Ishmael 'because he is your offspring' (21.13). So Abraham provides food and water and sends her away leading the lad by the hand. The story has a happy ending – the Lord *was* kind to the lad Ishmael: he lived in the wilderness of Paran, became an expert with the bow and eventually married a woman from the land of Egypt. He did indeed have twelve sons.

Assisted Reproductive Medicine

The collaboration of an Oldham gynaecologist, Patrick Steptoe, with a Cambridge embryologist, Bob Edwards, over many years showed that it was possible to take the eggs from a woman with blocked fallopian tubes, fertilize them in a dish outside the body, and then transfer them to her uterus, where they could implant and develop. At that time many thought this to be a very dangerous procedure.

Reproductive medicine has moved forward in leaps and bounds since that time and all levels of treatment have benefited from the precision which that work provided. IVF is an accepted procedure and over 160,000 babies have been born throughout the world as a result of IVF alone. There are few countries that do not provide some level of fertility treatment – that level will depend on their resources and priorities. It is probable that over 16,000 babies have been born as a result of cryopreservation and freezing of embryos. Several thousand babies have been born as a result of microinjection of sperm directly into the oocyte (egg).

Headlines in the press which herald each new development, and which talk about miracle babies, egg donation, surrogacy, microinjection etc., may raise the hopes of many childless couples whilst bringing pain to others for whom perhaps the technology has come too late, is unacceptable to them for personal or religious reasons, or for whom the new technology has not been successful –

even after over twenty years since the birth of the first 'test-tube' baby, treatment is much more likely to fail on each cycle than to succeed. Old wounds which they thought had healed are easily reopened and the 'bleeding' starts all over again. Each new development pushes out a sharp edge to highlight their failure. Human reproduction really does not work too well.

Childless couples are continually reminded of their plight. Everyday events such as shopping mean that they dodge the pushchairs and the prams, they rush past the shelves full of nappies, baby powder and baby food, and when they look into their back garden they see a washing line empty of all but adult clothes.

Many people have felt that this new technology would open the floodgates to abuse, that science is going too far, that assisted reproductive medicine was interfering in a very personal area of our lives and separating the act of love from the moment of conception. But conception is not a moment – it is a process. It takes several days. For the first three days the embryo shows the biochemistry of the egg: the genes from the sperm are not expressed until the third day. The Human Fertilisation and Embryology Act (1990) recognized this when it stated:

1.-(I) In this Act, except where otherwise stated:

> Embryo means a live human embryo where fertilisation is complete.

> References to an embryo include an egg in the process of fertilisation, and for this purpose, fertilisation is not complete until the appearance of a two cell zygote.

Up to day 14 the embryo is a collection of identical cells, differentiation into different 'parts' of the body has not started and the embryo is able to split into twins, triplets and presumably quads. How can we talk about an individual, a person being created at the penetration of the sperm through the zona pellucida – the shell surrounding the oocyte (egg)? If we say that the soul, the person, starts as early as that, we also have to say that 60–70 per cent of persons, souls, never get anywhere, because 60–70 per cent of embryos never implant and something like 20–25 per cent of implanted embryos will miscarry.

The Roman Catholic Church, in its teaching published in 1986 and in subsequent years, has been very critical of modern reproductive medicine. They argue that to do anything which might injure the embryo is a violation, an abuse, against the person which that embryo represents, that nothing should be done which is not beneficial to that embryo itself. The technology has moved forward with a greater range of treatments emanating from an increase in our understanding of human reproduction – the success rate has improved. But the absolutist attitude of the Catholic Church is still as rigid.

Yet to assume that an individual comes about immediately after fertilization is taking too simplistic a point of view. The fertilized embryo has to develop, to hatch, to implant, to differentiate into a foetus, to proceed through gestation and has to be born, before an individual or person can move forward.

Many people are totally unaware of this poor success rate – for them their dreams of having a family are realized with little delay or difficulty. For others the monthly return to menstruation is a cruel reminder that something is wrong. Their friends and relatives seem to be breeding like rabbits all around them but they have failed. Those familiar words at their wedding service – from the Book of Common Prayer: 'We beseech thee, assist with thy blessing these two persons, that they may both be fruitful in procreation of children ... that they may see their children Christianly and virtuously brought up'; or in the words of the Alternative Service Book 1980: 'Bless this couple in the gift and care of children' – seem so hollow now.

The early research allowed IVF to become a reality, and continuing research will make even more dreams come true. But it needs to be controlled research. And it is the intent of that research which is so important, and that intent must have a realistic chance to improve methods of contraception, to advance the treatment of infertility, or to help in the understanding of genetic disease.

Where Did I Come In?

I first became involved in this area of medicine almost by accident. I had joined the teaching staff in the Physiology Department of

Cambridge University, in 1970 teaching cell biology. By chance my room was on the fifth floor, just around the corner from Bob Edwards. Our areas of teaching overlapped and, because there was no adequate lift in those days, we frequently met on the stairs. Simple comments – 'It's a nice day', or 'I see you have had a hair cut' – soon turned to discussions of the implications of the work which Bob Edwards had started with Patrick Steptoe a year or so earlier.

In 1973 I had completed my theological training and was ordained an Anglican priest and our conversations on the stairs turned to discussions on the possible ethical implications of their work and then, after the birth of the first IVF baby in 1978, to the practical implications. In 1981, after the founding of Bourn Hall Clinic I was invited, by Steptoe and Edwards, as an Anglican priest and scientist, to be a founding member of an ethics committee to guide that clinic. There were no guidelines in existence at that time and that committee of five independent people was asked to look critically at the technology, to formulate guidelines to cover all the existing possibilities and to look forward to future developments which were on the horizon. They met at two-monthly intervals. That committee continues today and still feels that a Christian voice is essential in its deliberations.

Legislation

The Government set up the Warnock Committee in 1982, which reported back in 1984. The ethics committee contributed to their work and responded to their findings to the Government. The Warnock Report put forward many proposals for controls and regulations which it was felt were necessary in the light of this rapidly advancing field of medicine. It argued that research on human embryos should be allowed up to 14 days – with a dissenting view from three of its members, who felt that research on human embryos should be banned – and also proposed that surrogacy should be banned – with two dissenting voices.

The concerns which society showed towards the new reproductive technology resulted in many debates and arguments and many private members' bills being introduced in Parliament. The Enoch Powell Unborn Child Protection Bill, introduced in 1985, would have banned all research on human embryos and would have required childless couples to seek permission from the Secretary of State for Health before proceeding with treatment, and such permission would have been valid for only three months. The 'Right to Life' lobby was very strong and the feeling in 1985 suggested that a large majority was heavily in favour of banning research. A counter lobby group, 'Progress', took up the challenge. In the event a vote was never taken and the bill failed on procedural grounds.

Several other Members of Parliament reintroduced the Unborn Child Protection Bill but, in spite of strong and often very emotional support, all were defeated in filibuster moves.

It was not until 1990 that the Human Fertilisation and Embryology Act was passed – one of the most comprehensive pieces of legislation to cover assisted reproductive medicine anywhere in the world. Some of the major parts of that Act were:

- to set up the Human Fertilisation and Embryology Authority (the HFEA). This Authority would have statutory powers to control and regulate certain aspects of assisted reproductive medicine. Over the years it has drawn up a very useful code of practice which all licensed clinics must observe, and provides information to patients about individual clinic success rates. All clinics have to undergo an annual inspection by the Authority.

- to license treatment, storage and research. Initially Parliament was asked whether it wished to license treatment and storage (Clause 11 (2)) or treatment, storage and research (Clause 11 (1)). The vote in both houses was strongly in favour of Clause 11 (1) which allowed research but limited it to 14 days – defined with prohibitions in Schedule 2 of the Act. Some people feel that while the Act is one of the most comprehensive regulatory Acts in the world it is also the most permissive in that it allows for regulated research and freezing of embryos. Some countries have banned research on human embryos and severely restrict the freezing and storage of embryos.

- to define who is the mother and who is to be considered as the father in donor-assisted treatments. Section 27 defined the mother as the woman who carried and gave birth to the child, and section 28 defined the father as her husband/ partner. Thus registration of children born as a result of donor-assisted treatments is as for any other child.

- to allow for surrogacy and define procedures to provide for a change in parentage, necessary because of the definition of mother in section 27.

- to set limits on the storage of gametes and embryos (section 14). Gametes may be stored for ten years and embryos for five. This has been amended (1996) to allow for storage to ten years in certain circumstances. If after that time they have not been 'used', donated to another couple or donated for research they must be destroyed. This places a moral burden upon the embryologist who must by statute undertake that destruction.

In August 1996 the first five-year-limit period of storage under the Act came into effect. Many couples had not kept contact with the clinics and in the absence of proper consent for donation or extension the embryologist under the Act had to destroy several thousand embryos. Why could they not be 'adopted'? The law is quite specific in insisting that donation, for research or for the treatment of others, can only take place with full informed consent – no such consent had been given. Society expressed its horror at this imposition but under the law there was no alternative.

Most couples will need all the embryos they can get for their own treatment because, even today, the mean clinical pregnancy rate is only about 17.5 per cent and the mean live birth rate 13.2 per cent for each treatment cycle, with only slightly lower figures for frozen embryos. So realistically the chances of failure are much greater than the chances of success.

Many thousands of embryos are now in storage – a recent estimate suggests 500,000 worldwide. Even if only 10 per cent of these eventually could become babies, this represents 50,000 living entities that are kept in suspended animation – a thought that worries many people. Some couples will reject the freezing option because they do not want to be faced with making difficult decisions if and when they find that they no longer need them. The extension of storage from five years to ten will delay decisions even further, unless couples can be given time to face the alternatives *before* giving consent to freezing. Others feel that if you cannot guarantee that the embryos will not be damaged, you should not subject them to a 'hurtful' process and they therefore reject an option which might be beneficial to their chance of success.

Case 1

A couple had approached Bourn Hall Clinic for fertility treatment but had expressed reservations about some of their 'perceived' impressions about IVF. They were practising Roman Catholics and had been warned by their parish priest that clinics would undertake research on, or freeze, their embryos as a matter of course. The receptionist suggested they might like to talk it over with me, explaining that I was an Anglican priest.

They were very clear in their own minds that they could not accept:

- research;
- freezing of embryos;
- selection of embryos.

I was able to reassure them that none of those would take place without their consent, but that they should understand that their insistence that only three eggs should be placed with the sperm could result in poor fertilization or none at all.

'Fine,' they said, 'we accept that, but we don't want there to be any chance of there being spare embryos for freezing. Neither do we want there to be any selection – that this embryo is better than that one!'

'That's all right,' I replied, 'but there is a condition which, although rare, does exist – that is when two sperm simultaneously penetrate the egg. This results in three packages of chromosomes instead of two and cannot develop normally – in fact it can produce a life-threatening situation called a hydertidform mole, and you shouldn't expect the embryologist to transfer such an embryo – that could be placing an unacceptable moral stricture on the embryologist.'

'Yes, we can agree to that,' they replied.

As it happened she had five eggs – three were put with her husband's sperm, all three fertilized, but she did not become pregnant. On a second occasion exactly the same happened, but this time she did become pregnant and had twin boys. They still keep regular contact, even ten years later.

There are, however, additional worries in the freezing and storage of embryos that need to be addressed. We have already referred to a statutory freezing/storage limit and those patients will have to make decisions about the fate of any 'surplus' embryos that may arise.

Case 2

A couple had been for treatment, and the woman was close to ovarian hyperstimulation syndrome – a condition in which the woman responds over-enthusiastically to the hormones administered to such an extent that not only does she produce many eggs but the change in blood consistency can affect the kidneys and liver. Transferring the embryos to the uterus usually compounds this dangerous situation. So all the embryos were frozen, her clinical condition stabilized, and she suffered no adverse effects.

Some time later they returned for transfer of three of the frozen embryos. She became pregnant and had two lovely twin girls. They decided that the family was large enough – but what to do with the 24 frozen embryos? Their first thought was that they would be continually looking at every child in the East Anglia area if they donated them to other couples – 'Is that one of ours? That girl looks very much like one of our girls', and so on. Perhaps, then, they should just allow them to die. I visited them in their home with their two little girls, who did look very much like both parents, and one could understand their dilemma.

What about donating them to other couples well away from East Anglia, say Manchester? That, they felt, was the answer. St Mary's Hospital Manchester, one of the few NHS fertility clinics in the country, was delighted to accept them – they have a three-year waiting list for donated embryos. They did not have the resources to be able to collect them from Cambridge but as I counsel for that clinic in surrogacy cases I was able to take the flask of 24 embryos up to Manchester on my next visit a few weeks later.

Some additional dilemmas in freezing

To give such a recipient couple a chance of success, most clinics would want to transfer three donated embryos. So clinics may only accept that donation provided there were three or more embryos – the law in the UK does not allow embryos from different sources to be mixed and transferred together. The offer of donated embryos in 'ones and twos' is usually rejected. The screening procedures required for donors (HIV, Hepatitis B and C, karyotyping, cystic fibrosis, VDRL etc.) can cost £600. Some couples who have had one or two embryos which they no longer need, or for whom there are strong clinical indications that it would now be dangerous to use them for their own pregnancies, wish to give those precious embryos a chance of a life (however small). Who will pay for the screening and perhaps transport of donations? Some patients have taken the very altruistic decision to pay for such costs themselves when faced with this dilemma.

We have already suggested that there may well be as many as 500,000 embryos stored in liquid nitrogen around the world. A large clinic such as Bourn Hall Clinic might well have as many as 9,000 embryos in storage and the number keeps rising. The number of embryos going into the freezer is greater than the number coming out. There is an imbalance in the technology – too many embryos are being created, compared with the number required for successful treatment for the patients from whom they came. The real dilemma is that it is not possible to tell which embryos will be successful, and we need to encourage the practitioners to move towards the point where satisfactory outcome of treatment can be achieved with fewer embryos so that fewer need to be frozen.

Hidden Dangers?

There is no evidence so far that the freezing of embryos, or injecting sperm directly into the egg, causes any increase in abnormalities when compared with IVF or the natural population. What is not known is whether any of the causes of infertility from the parents are transferred to the offspring. Until those children come to child-bearing age there will always be this uncertainty.

In this brief introduction to assisted reproductive medicine we recognize that successful treatment brings much joy into the lives of many infertile couples. But we must never forget the failure that may go with it – fertility treatment has a comparatively low success rate (average live birth rate per treatment cycle is still only about 15 per cent). Licensed research is directed to improving methods of treatment, just as the initial research brought about the birth of the first IVF baby in 1978.

In helping couples to be more completely human we must not forget the welfare of the child. The future child or children must be central in all our thoughts. It must be at the forefront of our minds. Finding solutions to one problem may indeed free us from one kind of distress only to impose others. What often seems to be a straightforward answer to a particular problem may have significant and far-reaching consequences for ourselves, our children and our families; that is something we cannot always foresee, and is one of the areas of implications counselling, which fertility clinics must now make available to all patients.

So, is assisted reproductive medicine interfering with creation? The developments of modern medicine and science are a part of an invitation to assist where nature has clearly failed. We are, if you like, co-creators in the act of creation and carry out our task with responsibility and with care.

At a meeting of the European Society for Human Reproduction and Embryology in Cambridge in 1987, Patrick Steptoe (1915–1988) introduced the following poem with these words: 'I wanted to put together some thoughts to show that doctors and scientists care, and that we share in the bereavement which the parents have.'

A TRIBUTE TO AN EMBRYO

This is a story about a very early embryo,
full of energy,
full of vitality
and full of potential.

Everything seems to be going fine,
then,
the chromosomes stop marching,
the spindles disintegrate

63

degeneration occurs
and the embryo dies.

SO SMALL AND YET SO PRECIOUS
So small!
Just a few tiny cells.
That speck of life was all we had;
All we had hoped for;
All that we prayed for.

The embryo we had created
Had tried so hard
And struggled to survive;
But never did complete its implantation.

Yet still we grieve that death:
The loss was all too real.
For if all had progressed;
If that potential had been fully realized;
This would have been that child
We dreamed about.

Somehow in ways we cannot now define:
That entity of life is held in love,
In God's most tender care
To be a vital part of his creation.

TA, March 1997

Suggested Reading

Catholic Reports

Instruction on Respect for Human Life in its Origin and on the Dignity of Procreation: Replies to Certain Questions of the Day. London, Catholic Truth Society, 1986.

Response to the Warnock Report. London, Catholic Media Office, 1984. Document submitted by the Catholic Bishops' Joint

Committee in Bio-ethical Issues to the Secretary of State for Social Services.

On Human Infertility Services and Embryo Research. Document submitted by the Catholic Bishops' Joint Committee on Bio-ethical Issues to the Department of Health and Social Services, June 1987.

Government Publications

Report of the Committee of Enquiry into Human Reproduction and Embryology. (Chairman, Dame Mary Warnock. Presented by the Secretary of State for Social Services.) London, HMSO, Cm 256, November 1987.

Unborn Child Protection Bill. London, HMSO, 1985. (Introduced as a Private Member's Bill by Enoch Powell MP; defeated by filibuster tactics.)

The Human Fertilisation and Embryology Act (1990). London, HMSO, 1990. (The Act came into effect on 1 August 1990.)

Human Fertilisation and Embryology Authority

Annual Report of the Human Fertilisation and Embryology Authority 1993. London, HFEA (Paxton House, 30 Artillery Lane, London E1 7LS).

HFEA, *Code of Practice, Manual for Centres.* London, HFEA, 1991.

British Medical Association (BMA)

British Medical Association, *Report on Surrogacy 1990.* London, British Medical Association (Tavistock Square, London WC1H 9JP).

BMA, *Changing Conceptions of Motherhood: The Practice of Surrogacy in Britain.* London, BMA, 1996, ISBN 0 7279 1006 X.

Tim Appleton

My Beginnings – A Very Special Story. Cambridge, The IFC Resource Centre (44 Eversden Road, Harlton, Cambridge CB3 7ET; e-mail: tca@ifc.co.uk; http://www.ifc.co.uk), 1996. (ISBN 1 873663 21 8) Tells the story of six variations of IVF for children.

I'm a Little Frostie. Cambridge, The IFC Resource Centre (see above), 1996. (ISBN 1 873663 51 X) Tells the story of frozen embryos for children.

Assisted Reproductive Medicine. Cambridge, The IFC Resource Centre (see above), 1996. An interactive CD-ROM which looks at many facets of the new technologies.

Assisted Reproduction: Two Decades of Progress. Cambridge, The IFC Resource Centre (see above), 1999. An interactive CD-ROM in which the author looks back at the last 20 years with key experts from around the world, and looks forward to developments on the horizon. In two volumes:
Vol. 1: Clinical and scientific.
Vol. 2: Legal, ethical, social.

Other

My Story (DI [Donor Insemination] Support, Dept of Obstetrics and Gynaecology, Jessop Hospital, Sheffield.

D. Morgan and R.G. Lee, *The Human Fertilisation and Embryology Act 1990: Abortion and Embryo Research, the Law.* London, Blackstone Press Ltd, 1991.

CHAPTER SIX

Euthanasia and Assisted Suicide

Michael Langford

Some Distinctions and Clarifications

When people discuss the rights and wrongs of euthanasia a lack of clarity respecting words tends to confuse the debate. Let us begin, therefore, by looking at the term 'euthanasia', and see how it relates to 'assisted suicide'. Literally, 'euthanasia' comes from two Greek words and simply means 'good death'. In normal usage, however, the word is restricted to cases of the deliberate killing of *other persons* for the sake of their good, or alleged good. Thus it is distinguished from 'suicide', which is the deliberate killing of oneself, even if this is for one's believed good, and from 'assisted suicide', which is the helping of someone else to commit suicide, even if this is believed to be a 'good death'.

Despite these common distinctions, discussions of euthanasia and of assisted suicide tend to merge into each other, and it is easy to see why. Consider the example of Jane, who is likely to go into a coma from which she may never wake and who asks me to make sure that when the coma begins she is able to die quickly. This can be achieved either by insisting that no 'heroic' treatment is used, or by taking some more positive step, such as the giving of a lethal injection. Her motives are two: first, a desire not to be a burden on others, and second, a wish to avoid what she regards as an undignified, drawn-out death. Technically, giving the injection would be classed as 'euthanasia' or as 'active euthanasia'. The avoidance of life-saving treatment would be called 'passive euthanasia' by some, and 'letting die', or some variation of this, by others. In both circumstances, if I regard myself as Jane's agent, who is merely carrying out her orders, then it might be argued that these situations are 'really' cases of assisted suicide.

However, it should be noted that the term 'passive euthanasia', as commonly used, covers two situations which, according to some people, need to be sharply distinguished. The first is when the intention of the withdrawal of treatment is the death of the patient, the second is when the intention is 'to let nature follow its course', and the *result* is death. Others, as we shall see, deny the validity of this distinction, and others again deny any real distinction between 'killing' and 'letting die'.

From a *legal* perspective the responses to euthanasia and assisted suicide, and their relationship to each other, are fairly clear. The giving of a lethal injection to an unconscious patient in the foregoing circumstances would be called 'euthanasia', and is illegal in almost all countries. (Holland has a system where, provided a certain protocol is followed which includes the use of two physicians, cases of active euthanasia will not be prosecuted. The state of Oregon is proposing legislation to a similar effect. The Northern Territory of Australia passed a law in 1996 allowing for euthanasia in certain situations, but this law was later revoked.) Allowing Jane to die by refusing life-saving treatment would be mandated when there is a legally binding 'living will' to this effect. Where there is no such directive the situation is more complex, but the refusal to treat would be legal if a good argument could be made that the proposed treatment was essentially 'futile'. In other words, what some call 'passive euthanasia' is generally allowed, whether or not the intention is the death of the patient, as the judicial decisions in the 1993 British case of Tony Bland illustrated. Meanwhile (unassisted) suicide is now legal. However, the overall legal situation is complicated by the fact that sometimes juries will refuse to bring in a conviction for (illegal) euthanasia or assisted suicide if they are sympathetic to the accused, regardless of the evidence. Also, authorities are sometimes not eager to bring these matters to trial. The cases of suicide allegedly assisted by Dr Jack Kevorkian in the US bear witness to this.

Morally, however, the situation is much less clear. People disagree strongly over the ethics of both euthanasia and assisted suicide regardless of what the law dictates. With regard to what the law *ought* to dictate or allow, some feel that if suicide has been made legal, then 'assisted suicide' ought also to be legal, especially for people who find it difficult to achieve their own painless death, perhaps through physical incapacity. Some feel this assistance should not be limited to cases when the person is conscious, as in my example of Jane, and therefore they advocate the legalization of euthanasia.

The last paragraph illustrates an important complication. There are really two kinds of moral question at issue. The first can be called the 'strictly moral' issue – which is whether or not euthanasia or assisted suicide can ever be 'right'. The second can be called the 'moral-legal' issue – which is whether or not euthanasia or assisted suicide ought to be legal in certain circumstances. It is important to see that the latter is a different moral question from the first, since if it is agreed that something is immoral it does not necessarily follow that it should be illegal. In this paper I shall reflect on both the strictly moral and the moral-legal issues, but the latter is the more urgent. The reason for this is that in the case of the strictly moral question intelligent people may continue to disagree, and although the results of this disagreement may be serious, society often has to live with such disagreements. In the latter case, although individual citizens may continue to disagree, society *has to make a decision*. Either the law will, or will not allow these things, and clarity about what is legal is essential.

Before we look at what I have called the strictly moral question some further clarifications are necessary. If Jane is conscious, then we must assume that any assistance in suicide is voluntary, or our position becomes immediately untenable. But suppose, unlike Jane, John has given no directive or other clear indication of wishes, and goes into a coma from which he is virtually certain not to wake. In such cases, when continued biological life seems 'futile', some people advocate either passive or active euthanasia. Other typical examples of where such action is recommended are those of a severely brain-damaged newborn who could not give consent, and of an elderly Alzheimer's patient who could have given consent, before the onset of the disease, but did not. In all of these cases people often use the terms 'involuntary' or 'non-voluntary' euthanasia. I shall use the term 'non-voluntary' because the term 'involuntary' suggests that the proposed euthanasia is not only without the patient's consent, but is actually contrary to their expressed wishes. (Since it is hard to see any justification for 'involuntary' euthanasia I shall not discuss it here.)

Clearly, non-voluntary, active euthanasia raises the greatest worries. In practice, when all treatment seems 'futile', many patients are 'allowed to die ' with little or no protest, but deliberate non-voluntary killing is regarded by many as exceedingly evil. However, there is a problem here because, as has already been indicated, the distinction between 'euthanasia' (in the 'active' sense) and 'letting die' is challenged by a number of writers, and it is necessary to look at this distinction before going further. Is it the case that 'letting die' is really different from deliberate killing? (On this matter see also Alistair Campbell, in Gill (ed.), pp. 86–8 [Suggested Reading].)

Those who deny the validity of the distinction argue that since the result of both is the same, namely the immediately or near immediate death of the patient, the use of the distinction simply masks what is really going on. Moreover, it is alleged that when we remove life-support systems, although we may not admit it, our intention is really the same as in the case of active euthanasia, namely the death of the patient. A third strand of the argument consists in a challenge to the distinction between 'heroic' or 'extraordinary' means of life support on the one hand, and 'ordinary' on the other. What may seem 'extraordinary' at one time, for example, when the very first antibiotics were on the market, might become standard treatment at another. This suggests that terms like 'heroic' are very imprecise, and once again, may be a way of masking what is really going on.

Despite these objections, the majority of those involved in the health professions feel that the distinction between killing and letting die is both legitimate and useful (although, of course, this does not necessarily prove that it is valid). The argument here can easily become very technical, so I shall only indicate the principal grounds for maintaining the distinction. First, it is often denied that the result of giving a lethal injection and of removing treatment is always the same. When life-support systems are removed, for example in a hospice for the terminally ill, death does not always follow nearly as quickly as expected. This fact, in turn, supports the claim that there really is a distinction between 'letting nature take its course' (which does not, in all circumstances, mean immediate or nearly immediate death), and 'killing'. It is for this reason that I agree with those who dislike using the term 'passive euthanasia' as a synonym for 'letting die'.

Those who support the validity of the distinction also counter-attack as follows. When people insist on continuing to give life support in virtually 'hopeless' cases, the intent, it is claimed, is not therapy (which is the normal end of medicine) but 'to prolong the dying process'. Refusing to do this, the argument goes on, is not 'intending death', but 'intending the overall well-being of the patient'. Finally, even though the distinction between 'ordinary' and 'extraordinary' treatment may sometimes be vague, some precision can be given, in particular by those who make living wills. For example, there is a real distinction between feeding by spoon, which an ordinary member of a family is often able to provide, and an 'invasive' procedure, such as the use of a feeding tube, which can only be done with the help of technical expertise.

The Moral Question

Discussing the moral questions of euthanasia and assisted suicide, apart from any legal considerations, is somewhat artificial since what the law has to say on these matters actually affects the strictly moral question. The reason for this is that when a law forbids something, especially when that law has been made by a democratic process, this by itself provides a moral reason for not doing it, since there is, in general, a moral duty to obey the law. This 'reason' is not absolute, for there can be extreme situations where a moral person can believe that they ought to break a law which they hold to be grossly unjust, but in democratic societies these situations are rare. Nevertheless, let us try to answer the questions 'Could euthanasia, and could assisted suicide be morally justified – apart from questions of legality?'

There are two principal grounds on which a positive answer is given, and in this paper I shall restrict my comments to these.

The first relies on the principles of 'autonomy', according to which there is a moral duty to allow people to use their own judgements concerning what they will do, and how they will be treated, except in the following circumstances: (i) they propose to do something that will directly hurt another person, (ii) they are not 'competent', for example, because they are too young or too mentally impaired to make crucial decisions. Both of these restrictions warrant long discussions, for example, about what kind of 'hurt' should be prevented and what exactly makes someone 'incompetent'. However, it is easy to see how a defence both of euthanasia and of assisted suicide can be based on the principle of autonomy so long as certain safeguards are in place. (Virtually no one is suggesting that healthy people going through a period of depression should be assisted in either way.) In the case of rational persons who want to make fundamental decisions concerning their own lives, surely, it is argued, we need some compelling reason to say no. If we add to this a general principle to the effect that we ought to help other people to achieve their wishes, then there is a clear case for voluntary euthanasia and for assisted suicide.

The second argument relies on the principle that we should, whenever possible, reduce suffering. In the case of someone asking us to assist in suicide, then we can assume that there is extreme mental suffering, even if physical suffering is at least partially under control by drugs. Assisting people in such cases might then seem reasonable, or even demanded. In the case of those who are unable to express their wishes and who face physical or mental suffering, then 'helping them out of their misery' seems a natural consequence of the same principle. In this case, however, not only voluntary euthanasia might be justified, but also non-voluntary euthanasia. When someone is actually in a coma there may be no suffering (although there is, in fact, some debate on this matter, because we do not fully understand the workings of the unconscious mind), but there is certainly suffering experienced in anticipation of such a state.

On the contrary side there are again two principal arguments, plus a third one that applies especially to health professionals.

The first is sometimes called the 'sanctity of life' argument. The term 'sanctity of life' is notoriously vague, especially since few of its most ardent supporters believe that we should do everything to preserve merely biological life in *all* circumstances. For example, when an anencephalic baby ('baby K', born without the upper part of the brain) was kept alive for more than a year as a result of a decision by the highest court in Virginia, almost all agreed that this was an exercise in futility. However, when stated in less than absolute terms – as a claim to the effect that human life should be given huge respect, even if this means great inconvenience – then there is much to be said for such a principle. It would seem to underlie, for example, much of our concern for human rights. The argument can then be developed as follows: if we wish to encourage respect for life in all areas, including our respect for starving and inpoverished people all over the world, then we need to have extraordinary justification either for deliberately taking life, or for not doing all we can to preserve it. Since modern analgesics can prevent almost all cases of physical pain, it is better, therefore, to err on the side of maintaining life, and not to co-operate in the decision of others to end their lives.

The second argument is based on the need to protect the vulnerable. Let us suppose that euthanasia and assisted suicide become generally acceptable, and that a certain grandfather Billy Jones is in expensive long-term care. It is subtly (or perhaps not so subtly) suggested to him that in staying around, and not 'ending' things now (like his friends Barbara and Joe), he is really being selfish. In addition to the financial costs, precious resources are being tied up. Now, what is meant to be a purely voluntary decision (if it be a proper decision at all), has become subject to pressure. Many health workers are extremely worried about this prospect, and of hundreds of possible variations on it, and believe it would be impossible to develop adequate safeguards. Better then to continue the present rejection of euthanasia and assisted suicide, especially in the light of the development of modern analgesics for those who suffer. (On this matter of protecting the vulnerable see also Gill (ed.), pp. 53, 63, 94; see Suggested Reading.) This argument is often combined with an appeal to enlarge the provision of palliative care, which in many cases has helped to make the final days of dying people much less stressful.

The third argument concerns the 'Hippocratic' tradition of health professionals, and more specifically the Hippocratic oath which used to be taken by doctors and which forbids both euthanasia and assisted suicide. The tradition has been so closely allied to the enhancement and preservation of life that to include within it a systematic practice of terminating life seems to many to involve a dangerous undermining of it.

It should be noted that none of these arguments, on either side of the debate, are 'knock-down' arguments that settle the matter one way or the other. All of them are rather arguments that seek to balance competing principles (like respect for autonomy and respect for human life), and to suggest that the weight of the argument lies one way rather than another. This, I suggest, is usually the appropriate way to argue when we are dealing with controversial issues in which it is well known that equally intelligent and well-meaning people come to different conclusions. It does not suggest that there are not other issues (such as the torture of political prisoners) where we are dealing with 'absolute' wrong, rather than, as here, the balancing of arguments, and the balancing of moral principles that are sometimes in tension with each other. If one holds that there is a single, overarching moral principle, as utilitarians do, then there is in theory a 'right' answer to each moral dilemma; the problem is simply that we may not be able to discover it. However, if, like myself, one believes that there may be several independent moral principles (like autonomy and justice), then in many cases there *is* no single 'right' answer, however hard we think. There is instead the need to make a creative decision.

This 'pluralist' position is quite different from 'relativism' as normally understood. In relativism there may be no 'really' right *or* wrong answers. If there are 'real' moral principles – as I suggest – then there are frequently 'real' wrong answers, and only sometimes no single 'right' answer – that is, when genuine moral principles are in tension with each other. Another point to stress is that this absence of a single 'right' answer when there is a conflict of moral principles is in what might be called 'the public domain'. Privately, because of my individual gifts, my previous commitments, and my prayer life, there may be only one thing that is right 'for me'.

The Moral-Legal Question

When we ask whether the law should continue to disallow euthanasia and assisted suicide, the relevant arguments are similar to the foregoing, but with a new twist. If it is felt that these things are morally acceptable, then there would seem to be an over-whelming case for legalization. However, if there are serious doubts about their moral wisdom, the situation is less clear.

Let us assume that one feels, as I do, that the balance of the moral argument is against the morality of euthanasia and of assisted suicide (for all three of the reasons I have given), then, as we noted earlier, it does not necessarily follow that these things should continue to be illegal. It is not the role of law to forbid and sanction all the things we hold to be wrong. To do so would be to move towards a 'moralistic' system of law that most of us would consider to be in conflict with individual liberty. A more moderate view, based on a famous argument by J. S. Mill, is that the law should only forbid those immoral things that directly hurt others.

At this point we could easily be involved in a long debate about the kinds of 'hurt' from which it is necessary to protect people by law. If we include any psychological hurt, then people can use their hurt feelings, whatever they may be, in a kind of blackmail, to prevent others from doing a whole range of things that are important for their sense of well-being. However, one strand of the previous moral argument against both euthanasia and assisted suicide refers to what might be called a 'strong' example of 'hurt'. If vulnerable people are pressured to terminate their lives in a way that makes their decisions less than fully voluntary, serious harm has been done to them. This is one ground on which a powerful case can be built for maintaining a legal ban on both active euthanasia and assisted suicide. This position can be given added strength by pointing out that in cases of human experimentation, it is universally accepted that participation must be 'voluntary', and this excludes using 'captive populations', like prisoners or medical students. The reason for this is that such populations are likely to be 'pressured' to give a consent that is less than voluntary. (The ban on human experimentation on the very young or the mentally incapacitated is not absolute. When the potential benefits are great, the risks minimal, and appropriate 'proxy' consent is obtained, some paediatric research, for example, is allowed. This is an example of balancing the competing principles of 'doing no harm' (to the experimental subject) and of 'doing good' (to others).)

When the issue of voluntariness is taken into account, then the single most important question in the legalization debate is whether or not sufficient safeguards can be built into any proposed legislation to give adequate protection to the vulnerable. I am one of those who have serious doubts about this, and this is why, even though I do not claim to provide a 'knock-down' argument, I am still against substantial changes in the law on these matters. An additional argument for this conclusion will emerge in the last section.

The Christian Perspective

In view of the general theme of this book, readers may be surprised that so far there has been no explicit use of particularly Christian arguments, and only one reference to prayer. The reason for this is that when we discuss a particular ethical issue, most Christians take the view that what is right and wrong for them is also what is right and wrong for all human beings. This seems to be the import of St Paul's teaching in the second chapter of Romans when he claims that gentiles, who do not know the law of Moses, have, nevertheless, a moral law 'written in their hearts'. It follows that if Christians believe that (say) euthanasia is wrong, they believe it is wrong not just for them, but for all people. But if this is the case, we ought to be able to give reasons for the wrongness of euthanasia that do not depend on either the Bible or Christian tradition, both of which may be either unknown, or even positively rejected as guides by many of those with whom one discusses the issue.

However, if it is agreed that there is a common content to Christian ethics and human ethics, it does not follow that the Bible and Christian tradition have nothing important to add. What is added, I suggest, can be summarized under three headings, grace, the status of moral principles, and special content.

Grace

It is one thing to believe that a certain action is morally right, another thing to have the strength always to perform it. Christianity teaches doctrines of forgiveness and enabling grace which, it is held, makes it more possible for people actually to do what is right.

The status of moral principles

If we believe that moral values flow, not only from human conventions and aspirations, but from the loving purposes of God in creation, then morality is given a significance that, in my view, it cannot have for the atheist, however morally good the atheist may be. Psychologically, belief in a purposive order behind and within the world we see gives morality a special importance and sense of urgency. It gives force to the idea of moral 'discovery'.

Special content

Although, following St Paul, we may hold that the content of ethics is basically the same for all human beings, there can be special cases where particular Christian values make a difference. In addition to this, Christianity, like the other great religious traditions, may often be able to 'blaze a trail'. That is to say, it may highlight important values *before* these values come to be generally recognized by people all over the world.

In the light of the foregoing, let us consider whether there are special Christian values or insights that bear on the issues of euthanasia and assisted suicide. Two suggestions come to mind.

First, the belief that we have a particular vocation from God, which only we can fill, has led Christians – as well as many other monotheists – to have added reasons for rejecting suicide, and therefore euthanasia and assisted suicide as well. However, some caution is needed here, for there are different kinds of suicide. There are rare cases of people committing suicide, not for their own sakes, but for the sake of others. For example, they may kill themselves rather than fall into enemy hands while holding information that is vital for the survival of their friends. In such cases, since we may believe that we are unable to withstand torture, I for one do not think that suicide is wrong, even though the Christian tradition has usually been absolutist about this. It is interesting to note, too, that when Kant gives his famous argument to the effect that suicide is wrong, he actually argues that suicide 'for the sake of one's own good or convenience' is wrong – and then concludes (I think erroneously) that he has proved all suicide to be wrong. Never-theless, outside such rare circumstances, Christians are likely to believe that however hopeless circumstances seem, God can use their lives for some purpose – be it prayer, or example, or comfort to others. This consideration applies especially to our requests for assisted suicide, but even when we are likely to become un-conscious, some Christians think this provides an additional reason for refusing to ask for euthanasia.

Second, there is the belief that suffering, while not itself a good, can be the means for bringing about good, as in the supreme example of the cross. Since most cases of requests for either euthanasia or assisted suicide are in order to avoid suffering of some kind, a Christian is more likely to believe that the suffering, if unavoidable except by these means, may be something which can be used for some good, even if this is simply the spiritual purification of one's own soul.

I think that there is force in both of these suggestions, but I would add two cautions. The first is that neither of them seems to me to provide grounds for 'continuing the dying process'. In other words, they provide added grounds for being hesitant about active euthanasia and assisted suicide, but not for the decision to 'let nature take its course'. The second is that it is one thing for me to choose to live because of a belief in vocation, and quite another thing to demand this of others. Even more, it is one thing to decide to accept suffering for oneself, but quite another thing to choose suffering for another. I suggest, therefore, that for the Christian, while both arguments provide additional grounds in respect to the 'strictly moral questions', they do not add to the grounds for the 'moral-legal' questions regarding euthanasia and assisted suicide. Particularly in a pluralistic society such as ours (but arguably in any society), the imposition of specifically Christian views should be resisted. I am still against the legalization of euthanasia and assisted suicide, but on grounds that I hold to be essentially independent of my Christian beliefs, including my beliefs about vocation and the redemptive power of suffering.

Living Wills

In many parts of the world, including most American states and Canadian provinces, people while conscious can make what are called 'living wills' (in the US) and 'advance health care directives' (in Canada), which mandate what treatments one will have *after* one ceases to be mentally competent. Certain limitations are built into the laws, for example, one cannot ask for anything illegal, and one cannot *demand* any treatment – for example, if it be considered futile, or too expensive for the State to provide. However, one can demand that in a variety of circumstances treatment be discontinued, even if this means that one dies.

Similar legislation is being considered for the United Kingdom. At present, in this country, one can make a living will, and it may influence one's treatment when one ceases to be conscious, but there is no legal necessity that it should. Frequently the decisions of relatives are accepted, even if they are contrary to the wishes of the patient. Such legislation has a bearing upon euthanasia and assisted suicide, especially since the termination of 'treatment' may include the use of any artificial nutrition or hydration. But if hydration is discontinued nearly all patients die within about five days – not simply through thirst, but because of an imbalance in essential electrolytes.

There is a complication here in that 'treatment' is an ambiguous term. In America, courts have sometimes ruled that giving fluids by a tube is a kind of 'treatment' while a recent court in the United Kingdom determined otherwise. What matters, therefore, is that anyone making a living will should be specific about this crucial question, and indicate when, if at all, they want all hydration discontinued.

In my view the foregoing provides an additional argument for rejecting calls for the legalization of euthanasia and assisted suicide. One of the grounds that make the cases for these things plausible is the picture of people being forced to continue to live, whether conscious or unconscious, perhaps for months or years, in what they feel to be a worthless and undignified way. But in fact, given living will legislation, anyone can choose 'to let nature take its course', even if this means that one will be dead within about five days, by insisting on no hydration now, and writing a living will that forbids it when coma sets in. In most of North America this is the true situation now. Therefore, the picture that is painted of a long-drawn-out process being forced on people is often quite misleading. Here I am not saying that such decisions are or are not moral (which would require much discussion), merely that the availability of living wills much reduces the force of arguments for the legalization of euthanasia and assisted suicide.

However, I do not want to suggest that this last point is an 'easy answer'. Dying through dehydration need not be a painful process for the patient (contrary to common belief), if they are in a typical end-of-life stage, and if proper 'mouth care' is provided. (I have this from experts in palliative care.) However, the process is often painful for the family, and for nursing staff who wish, quite naturally, to give water, at least by spoon, to patients who have resolutely said no. Also, some institutions are quite unprepared to allow such a process while a patient is in their 'care'. Further, only a small number of people, so far, have actually availed themselves of the opportunity to make living wills. Nevertheless, the potential of this legal instrument is huge, and indicates a realistic alternative to at least some of the problems that have led many thoughtful people to believe in euthanasia or assisted suicide.

My overall conclusion is that, on balance, I am not convinced of the need for legalizing either euthanasia or assisted suicide. There are arguments for these things that have merit, or 'weight', but the counter-arguments, especially those concerning respect for life, the protection of the vulnerable and the increasing provision of realistic alternatives (for example, with living wills), seem to me to be stronger.

There is one type of case, however, where I am unsure, and wonder whether special legal provision could properly be made. Modern pain killers, or 'analgesics', can deal with physical pain in all but very rare circumstances. However, such circumstances do occur, for example in Canada in the 'Latimer case', where adequate analgesics could not be given because they would have interfered with other drugs that were necessary for survival, and where the patient was not competent to refuse all treatment or make an advance health-care directive. In such rare circumstances, there could perhaps be some independent medical body that ruled on the question of whether extreme physical pain was unavoidable, and then make application to a court for special permission to use such massive doses of analgesic that the pain is removed, even if death occurs. The intent in such situations, as I see it, should be not 'death' as such, but the removal of physical pain. At present the law allows the giving of analgesics even if this will shorten life (as in the Annie Lindsell case in the United Kingdom), but this is interpreted in such a way that the massive doses needed to alleviate certain rare kinds of suffering are ruled out, since the death would follow almost at once.

Suggested Reading

T.L. Beauchamp and J.F. Childress, *Principles of Biomedical Ethics*, 4th edn. Oxford, Oxford University Press, 1994.

D. Cook, *The Moral Maze*, London, SPCK, 1983, Chapter 6.

R. Gill (ed.), *Euthanasia and the Churches*. London, Cassell, 1998.

J. Keown (ed.), *Euthanasia Examined*. Cambridge, Cambridge University Press, 1995.

T. Regan (ed.), *Matters of Life and Death*, 2nd edn. New York, Random House, 1986.

Index

The Society for Promoting Christian Knowledge (SPCK) was founded in 1698. It has as its purpose three main tasks:

- **Communicating the Christian faith in its rich diversity**
- **Helping people to understand the Christian faith and to develop their personal faith**
- **Equipping Christians for mission and ministry**

SPCK Worldwide serves the Church through Christian literature and communication projects in over 100 countries. Special schemes also provide books for those training for ministry in many parts of the developing world. SPCK Worldwide's ministry involves Churches of many traditions. This worldwide service depends upon the generosity of others and all gifts are spent wholly on ministry programmes, without deductions.

SPCK Bookshops support the life of the Christian community by making available a full range of Christian literature and other resources, and by providing support to bookstalls and book agents throughout the UK. SPCK Bookshops' mail order department meets the needs of overseas customers and those unable to have access to local bookshops.

SPCK Publishing produces Christian books and resources, covering a wide range of inspirational, pastoral, practical and academic subjects. Authors are drawn from many different Christian traditions, and publications aim to meet the needs of a wide variety of readers in the UK and throughout the world.

The Society does not necessarily endorse the individual views contained in its publications, but hopes they stimulate readers to think about and further develop their Christian faith.

For further information about the Society, please write to:
SPCK, Holy Trinity Church, Marylebone Road,
London NW1 4DU, United Kingdom.
Telephone: 0171 387 5282